Joyous
Every Day
Living

Joyous Every Day Living

HOW TO LIVE FULLY ALIVE... AND PARTY TILL CHECKOUT TIME!

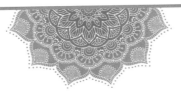

Beth Amine

Published by:
Beth Amine
www.joyouseverydayliving.com
joyouseverydayliving@gmail.com

Cover painting by Beth Amine
Cover and interior book design by Lynda Rae, Aurora Design Studio.
All paintings and quotes in this book are © Beth Amine.

First print edition published 2017
ISBN: 978-1979853453

To Patricia,

Thank you for the wonderful work you do in the world,

you are a great example of Joyous Living!

♥ Beth

CONTENTS

ACKNOWLEDGMENTS

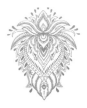

Nothing is accomplished without many hands, minds and hearts and I would like to acknowledge the people who have both contributed to this book and inspired all other areas of my life. My editor and friend, Andrea Warnecke was instrumental in seeing that the book was just right and got published. Lynda Rae, of Aurora Design Studio, is the graphic designer who made it so beautiful. My daughter, Yazmine Gingras reminds me to be fearlessly authentic and caring. I thank my sister and brother-in-law, Dida and Rich Merrill for their innovative thinking and for always taking the high road. To my story tellers, thank you for your candid and personal sharing. And lastly, to my friends and family who have given me constant support and encouragement, I am so happy to be celebrating this life with you. Enjoy!

—*Beth Amine*

Introduction

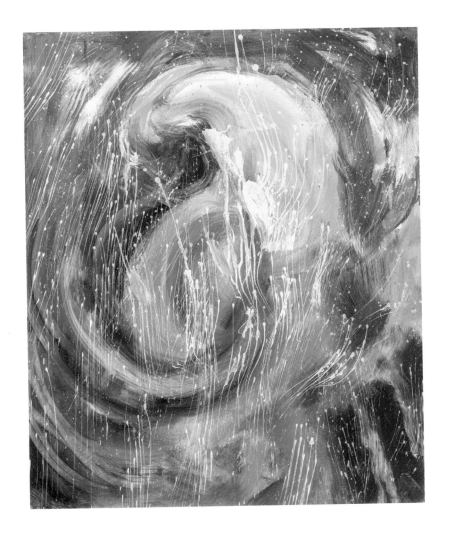

"I am a beautiful, eternal being of light moving through time."

Introduction

IT IS OUR ESSENTIAL NATURE to flourish. Joy and well-being are our natural state and purpose, yet so many of us find it challenging to maintain or even reach this fundamental condition. *Joyous Every Day Living* is a liberating, comprehensive how-to guide that offers a simple system for living happily in a state of perpetual health and rejuvenation. It encourages you to consistently choose fresh and expansive possibilities for creating deep, personal joy. This naturally overflowing enjoyment of life can then be shared with others.

Information that we constantly receive from a wide variety of external sources has a limiting message about our potential for creating a long and vibrant life. Our cultural paradigm insists that in the aging process, we must have an inevitable physical and mental decline. Yet we have the authority to consciously alter our expectations and generate our own positive outcomes. Often asking "What do I want?" and "What makes me feel good?" keeps us centered in answers that are the best choices for our individual lives.

This book is designed as a framework of support and inspiration for connecting to your own power and then choosing for yourself the habits that create consistent joy and vitality. It shows how to develop lifestyle choices that will keep you constantly thriving. We will explore what makes you feel the ecstasy of being alive and learn how to align to that place consistently. In other words, "Party till checkout time!"

Joyous Every Day Living is a dedication to embracing what it takes to fully actualize the enjoyment and wonder of each day. It is created from my experiences, explorations and observations in a life-long quest for self-knowledge, personal growth and the desire to deeply appreciate each moment of the gift of life.

I have spent the last 45 years as a professional artist. In making my living with art, I have painted, designed, performed, danced and written on a daily basis. However, my deep passion for self-exploration was always only part of the equation. Early on in my career, I began teaching visual art and dance movement with the desire to share the gifts of artistic expression with others. My current calling is focused on making the art experience accessible for everyone through movement videos, shrine making kits, inspirational imagery and writings. Around 2010, my reach expanded into the senior community and I saw first-hand how America is aging. As a member of the Baby Boomer generation which is defined in part by not wanting to grow old, I have included in this book a new approach to prevailing systems which has worked successfully for me personally. With expansive new possibilities, rejuvenation and aliveness can replace old concepts of how we must live out our lives.

Scientific research is also starting to confirm this shift with similar findings. Over the past 75 years, scientists have been redefining their assumptions about the way the world works and our place in the Universe. Older, separating, mechanistic views are being replaced with holistic quantum models. These new outlooks are included here to represent another point of view and corroborate the practical, mystical and spiritual content of this book.

Maintaining health and happiness at any age is a continuously evolving practice. Understanding and living with this creative process is for the courageous and the brave. Although there are many to help along the way, you are ultimately alone with your life, moving through the chaos of what is until you understand and embrace its artistic and liberating benefits. Comfort with ever-unfolding process has taught me much about the acceptance of current conditions as a way to the next best place. Although it can be extremely uncomfortable, as letting go and change can be, the ease and fluidity with life that it provides is priceless.

All of the practices outlined in this guide have come from a lifelong passion for self-knowledge and growth in order to allow more life in to be lived. The book is structured with each chapter being an aspect of aliveness that intertwines with all the others. The content for each quality is multi-layered, to provide a deeply embodied, internal experience. Every chapter begins with a quote and painting that are meant for personal meditation, inspiration and to visually and symbolically represent the essence of the chapter. Next are my thoughts on the subject, followed by personal experiences from a wide variety of people. Scientific confirmation on the spiritual and artistic content is then included. Finally, Practices show how to cultivate the different facets of aliveness for yourself. A blank note page is provided for your own explorations.

The base values of this guide are kindness to oneself and to others and the ability to experience the pleasure of life in all its permutations. The pervasive theme is connection to self and to others, together with the divine source and mysteries of life. Life is lived as an ever-unfolding, fun adventure of growth. All the chapters overlap and integrate. They are meant to provide alignment with the richness of the present moment, while experiencing self-acceptance and deepening personal potential. Yours is a beautiful journey and it is my absolute delight to be sharing these insights with you.

The seven most important points in this book are:

1. You are the ultimate authority in your life, the one to make the choices for yourself. You have the answers and the answers are yours to explore. Guidelines are contained here but the exact program is up to you.

2. Do whatever it takes to love yourself unconditionally. You are a unique and remarkable individual like no other.

3. Decide to feel good as your ultimate expression. Life is supposed to be pleasurable, and the now moment is all there is. Let's party!

4. Be appreciatively fulfilled with what is as your desires unfold. Then give undivided attention in the now to what you prefer.

5. Your thoughts are the blueprint for your reality.

6. Maintain a devotion to the sensual experience of life.

7. Allow your heart to lead.

If you would like to include your own story of growth, please send it to me via my blog site at www.joyouseverydayliving.com. We love to share!

MY STORY

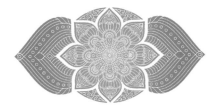

Writing this book was an enormous pleasure for me. It provided a fun opportunity to combine different languages of expression. With words and images, I was able to give you, from my heart, an experience of liberated spirit through my favorite forms of happiness: art, community and celebration.

My personal journey with art as an access to deep inner knowledge and strength began when I was a child growing up in multi-cultural Los Angeles. In a huge expansive world, my life was one of limitations and constricted self-expression. Family messages included, "The neighborhood is dangerous, don't go out."; "People are not to be trusted."; "There is not enough."; "That is not for you."; "You can't." All the classic inhibitors of joy! Yet all around me were inaccessible riches. Art-making became a way for me to experience freedom and a lavish inner life.

Post World War II Los Angeles provided a very poignant time for my coming of age. My large Baby Boomer High School class of over 700 students experienced the beginning of a massive cultural revolution - the Civil Rights Movement, Kennedy's assassination, the start of the Vietnam War and the arrival of the Beatles in America!

I finally left my neighborhood after the curfew was lifted in the 1965 Watts Riots and continued my education at UCLA and then

UC Berkeley. Majoring in Art and Literature, I was in the graduating class of 1968, which was at the epicenter of the social reinvention of the time. It was Party, Play and Think Outside the Box. Also inherent in the cultural history of this time was the idea of "taking it to the streets", which meant taking action on your beliefs. That model morphed for me into a positive practice of committed involvement with my community, both local and global. I arrived in lovely Santa Barbara in the early 1970s, finding a home after a year or two of unscripted nomadic travels.

It was in Santa Barbara, where I still live, that my deep explorations of spiritual and personal growth through the arts began. Along with my commissioned work, I also discovered my inner creative world through visionary paintings and inspirational writings. However, most art making is a solo pursuit and only involves the body in a way that serves it. Lifting ladders and paint cans, sitting for long periods at the computer to write, or using power tools for sculptures can be very physically demanding. I accessed my physical liberation through movement when I was in my mid 20's and serendipitously took a belly dance class, filling an unspoken need. I had emotional food issues at the time and was not at a healthy weight. Self-esteem and mind-body connections were missing from my life. I had to find the richness that lay beneath my self-doubt and pain from the past. A deep desire came to find a way to learn about this constriction, love it and release it to life that so I could expand. Dance provided this healing, and it has been a never ending source of delight in my life ever since my first class. All the arts united for me, creating a framework for the evolution of my own wholeness.

The subject of relationship or connection became a pervasive theme in all my work, as it is in this book. Uniting is the biggest path to joy, whether it is with our interior life or the world outside. Joy is my devotion and you are invited to the party!

Move

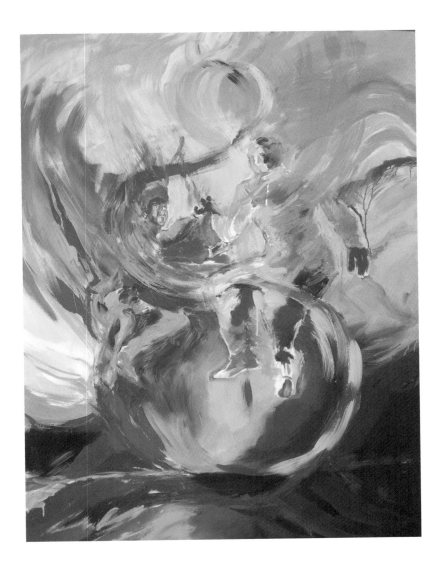

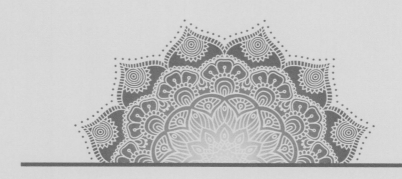

"*Dance was the first language
and immediately connects us to our source.*"

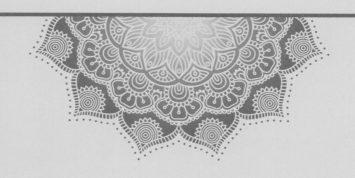

CHAPTER ONE

Move

JOYOUS EVERY DAY LIVING BEGINS with a focus on movement, one of the basic qualifying components of being alive. The act of moving reflects our essential natures, which thrive in a constant state of expansion. Our purpose is to open and grow in sync with the Universe we live in, as we are eternal life forms moving through time. Physical movement is crucial to well-being on all levels of our experience. It heals mind, body and emotions. Moving the body can be science, art, or even mystical experience. It is also the most primary way to create connection to self and the broader context of life.

Dance movement, which unites our physical awareness with music, is the oldest known ritual for linking to forces greater than oneself. Since early human history, people have moved to the rhythm of their heartbeat and simple percussion instruments to connect with and make sense of the vastness of experience.

Beyond its spiritual aspects, dance has been proven scientifically to be the number one activity for creating regeneration of brain cells and slowing the decline of mind and body. With consistent practice, agility, mobility and stability are sustained and the health of life-giving circulatory and respiratory systems can be maintained.

Simply put, dance is union. And most importantly, it is exhilarating fun!

I witness the miracles of movement constantly in my dance classes, which are for every level of fitness and cognitive ability. Individuals who did not smile, walk, or even lift their arms and breathe, come alive and vital when connecting their bodies to music. Others learn to shine and become unafraid to show up as who they essentially are.

Dance movement has the power to create a deep healing bond between our internal life and basic sense of value or feelings of worthiness. The theme of self-love is pervasive in this book as the essential component of both connection to feeling alive and to love and compassion for others. It is so beautiful and freeing to finally have the knowledge that we are worthy just because we are alive and therefore made of and from love. Creating a deep mind-body connection through music and movement roots this knowledge in our being. There is a profound unifying beauty in feeling all aspects of life through the sensuality of our physical experience.

The myth of scarcity and lack and therefore separation from the source of life goes very deep for us culturally. The thoughts that there is not enough or I am not enough are omni-present. One of the most challenging "not enoughs" for almost all of us is negative body judgment. Through movement, we join without thinking to our inner life and essential nature and can create complete freedom from this debilitating mind-set. Our thoughts create our reality. They can therefore create negative as well as positive conditions in our health and well-being. Dance is liberation into life-affirming choices.

STORIES

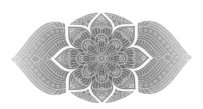

In my long career as a dance instructor, I have seen many experiences of profound change from the practice of dance movement. Eating disorders, self-loathing, physical conditions, addictions and inner fears have all been healed. Personally, dance has taught me much about the power and peace of total self-acceptance. After struggling for decades with judgment about my own looks and self-worth, one day I had the perception that I am fine the way I am. Imagine! It was mind-blowing and ground breaking. I looked in the mirror and had the usual personal and cultural perception that my body is not good enough. It needed more tone and less belly. Then I somehow clicked into the Now and was able to say: "I am perfect in my imperfections right now, the way I am. I am beautiful and in flux. I am the perfection of the Now Moment." It was a profoundly freeing experience. Pursuing the ideal image out there keeps us from what we seek, since it is a condition we are always moving towards but are never in. How painful it is to not accept our own unique beauty. What an easier, happier choice it is to just decide to feel good with ourselves as we are. This is where we find our own personal power, undiminished, through complete self-acceptance and self-appreciation. Our deepest inner nature of love matches our physical vehicle. The joy of dance movement helps us by-pass negative thoughts of self or body. It then allows the free flowing feeling of life's wholeness to be experienced until it becomes an embodied and consistent state. The opinions and biases of others then become completely unimportant. Remember, the relationship with your body is YOURS and yours alone!

Beyond possessions, a state of joy is the greatest achievement of success. And a good feeling body is the greatest factor for maintaining a continued state of joy and well-being.[1]

Delaney Harding

My name is Delaney and I am 17 years old. I am so excited to have the opportunity to share how dance has transformed my life.

I have had severe social anxiety and depression since I was 5. It wasn't until I was 11 and started dancing that I found my inner strengths and courage through dancing. For me, dance is highly therapeutic and is essential to me as breathing oxygen; for that, it is more effective than any medication. On the days when I struggled to get out of bed, I would get myself to my studio and let my body take control. Dancing transformed my outlook on life, my capabilities, and gave me a fresh mindset to take on the rest of the day. It is so liberating to feel in control and in tune with my body when the rest of the world is constantly changing and throwing obstacles in my direction. Over this past year, dance has taught me to be fearless in the pursuit of what sets my soul on fire.[2]

Lauren Breese

Dance has picked me up and put me back together more times than I can count. When my marriage failed, I set out to learn partner dancing. Lonely evenings turned into nights surrounded by people having fun while working up a sweat. I soon began exploring a variety of other dance genres that I had abandoned as a young adult setting out on a career path. At 40, I had rediscovered a creative outlet that quickly led to performing and choreographing.

But internally I was waging another battle. A corporate executive at a Los Angeles company, I was making more money than ever, working harder than ever and spending an enormous amount of time away from home. On the outside I was a successful businesswoman. Inside I was miserable and I knew I was not feeding my soul what it craved.

I earned my Yoga certification and was training in aerial dance while job stress sent my health into a tailspin. I didn't dance at all for almost a year. Then, a dance teacher asked me to substitute her class for a few months while she recovered from surgery. I instantly started feeling better. I resumed aerial dancing and quickly rediscovered how empowering and strengthening it was. Friends asked me to teach them, and soon I found myself starting a dance company.

In spite of life's heartbreaks, breakups and breakdowns, everyday I am reminded that dance is always my breakthrough to a healthier body and mind. Dancing "perfectly" is not the point of the journey. Every step of the way, dance teaches us how to take better care of ourselves and love ourselves more![3]

From Some of My Senior Joyous Movement Students:[4]

My doctor told me to see a physical therapist. I did and nothing happened. This class fixed it all! —ML

My back feels so much better after class. — CR

My pain from arthritis is relieved, I am so happy! —TW

I think every Grandmother should do this every day. It keeps us so alive. —HB

It reminds us of what we can still do. —YA

I come to class every week because it helps me think much more clearly! — GT

From an Alzheimer's and Dementia Day Care Staff Member:[5]

The group's mood is improved all the rest of the day. We wait all week for your Joyous Movement class! — SJ

Kathryn Eisler LeMay, PhD.

Observing Beth Amine conduct her Joyous Movement Class with the elderly population is inspirational.

As a clinical psychologist, I am impressed with her ability to combine activities that cause the spirits of geriatric clients to ignite. In addition, she is uniquely able to generate neuro-behavioral changes in one hour that are extraordinarily beneficial for any individual who has beginning to advanced stages of memory loss or balance impairment by her transformational methods of therapeutic exercise movement.[6]

Luciana Mitzkun, Dementia Care Specialist, Family Services Director, Friendship Center

While scientists are leaving no stone unturned in searching for a cure for Alzheimer's, regular physical still remains the only strategy proven to slow down the progression of cognitive loss associated with the disease.

Practicing regular physical exercise has been found to reduce risks and stave off the onset of Alzheimer's and dementia, another reason why all age groups should exercise. For people affected with cognitive impairment, however, exercising must also be fun.

That's why we are fortunate to have found Beth Amine! She is the creator of Joyous Movement, a program uniting music, dance, exercise, and memory training, that is also a lot of fun. People at every level of physical and cognitive ability benefit from participation in Joyous Movement. It is particularly beneficial for people with dementia, for whom activities options are increasingly limited. Patients suffering from dementia-related apathy come to life during Joyous

Movement classes. Beth keeps them smiling, engaged, and playfully active. They leave the classes uplifted and carry that positive feeling with them throughout the entire day. Beth's classes have been wonderful to our families affected with dementia and I hope she will continue assisting our community. She brings a bright shot of "can do" joy and optimism, so helpful to all who want to enhance and retain their cognitive abilities.[7]

SCIENCE

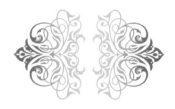

As my own maturity in life unfolds, I have been enjoying the radical concept that the older you get, the better you get. The body is pure energy that responds to our thoughts and the self-healing power of our co-operative cells is vast and natural. Yes, we can be in a self-induced state of rejuvenation and perpetual vitality with simple mental and physical practices.

Science is constantly confirming the validity of these new approaches. There is extensive research now on the benefits of movement, not just for physical fitness but also for subtler quality of life enhancements, including reduced anxiety and depression, as well as consistently better moods. Dance improves memory and cognitive functioning by using the mind in improvised decision-making which creates new neural pathways. Increased social interaction, non-verbal heart communication, improved self-esteem and confidence are more of its gifts.

Our brains are remarkably plastic, and will re-wire themselves and create new neural conduits when it is called for. We can stay younger for longer with greater cognitive (perception, memory, judgment, reasoning) storage. When we use our brains in new ways, we improve the synaptic or electronic communication between cells.[8]

I love that frequent dancing makes us smarter! Studies show (all the research is in the footnote section for your own further exploration) that of all physical activities, dance movement is the most effective way to preserve and restore cognitive skills and this was by a margin as big as 76%. This is because of the split-second decisions that dance requires and the variety of connections established when the mind is working with the body in joy and freedom. The brain is simultaneously coordinating mental, emotional and physical processes. Stimulating the mind through the body can prevent memory loss, while increasing sharper thinking.[9]

Just like the heart, the brain has its own rhythm. The internal cadences of the brain and nervous system appear to play an important role in everything, from walking to thinking. The rhythms of the brain begin with the firing patterns of individual brain cells. An abnormal rhythm can create a wide variety of physical conditions, such as tremors and other difficulties with movement. These symptoms are greatly reduced when individuals respond to the rhythms of music and dance. So make sure to keep moving and take a dance class often![10]

One of the basic discoveries of Quantum Physics is that atoms are not a physical structure made of separate particles, but are energy, a vibration. Therefore matter is energy, and our thoughts are very powerful in influencing matter. The observer of life has turned into a participant. The body is affected by the negativity or positivity of thought. New concepts say we are not victims of genetics either, but can influence this coded information as well. In this new scientific model, consciousness is a fundamental force in our Universe. Repeated, focused thought is the template that creates our reality. Our deep relationships with our bodies through the messages we constantly say to ourselves, allow us to take the power in maintaining good health. Coupled with the energy of our hearts, we materialize our life of choice. The combination of thinking and feeling allows manifestation to happen. This confirms the great personal power we have to take control of our own health and constant renewal as we uncover our true nature as expansive, creative multi-dimensional beings.[11]

PRACTICES

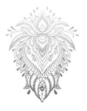

Get up and move all day! At least once an hour, get up from that computer, work or home obligation and take a few minutes for yourself. The number one hint is to breathe. Lift your arms above your head. Take a deep breath through your nose and exhale through your mouth as you lower your arms. Make noise if you can. Stretch to the sides, arms overhead, and just open your body up. Add a few gentle knee bends and shake from top to bottom. Just a few minutes taken regularly will make a huge difference in how you feel, your mental mood and sharpness, and help prevent that bottom half from getting chair spread. Keep your body happy, because if it is, you are!

Your body is pure energy and it is constantly responding to your thoughts. What if every negative and self-loathing thought manifested as disease in your energy field and then in the body? Instead, I find it enjoyable to pour love into each cell of my body as often as possible. This practice takes just a few minutes a day, and is time spent that is all for you. There are many visualizations available, or you can make up your own. See your body as a dancing whirl of golden light and your conscious essence as a white light. They are blending in a dance of mutual love. Or, choose whatever colors you like and radiate them on your body daily, any time of day, especially when you have a negative thought about the way it looks or feels. This is a communication with your body on its deepest levels. You can even visualize your DNA renewing!

Experience the pleasure of the body daily. Lavish it with good care. Take that bath, get that massage. And especially, listen to it. Instead of overriding the body's communications to you if you have an ache or pain, ask what this symptom is communicating about what is going on in your mental or emotional life.

Your body is the vehicle that carries you though this gift of the journey of a life that you have chosen to experience. And it was made to move. Include walking, bending and climbing in your everyday activities. I like to make my home or office my gym, doing leg stretches on book cases and arm push-ups on the sink. Walk up that neighborhood hill. Dance to one of your favorite songs every day. Just take those few daily minutes and put the music on. Just as important, drench your body with music daily.

Alternating styles of movement keeps it fresh. Yoga, weight-bearing exercise and expressive dance movement are all great and help round out your fitness program. I also highly recommend Belly Dance as an amazing, non-injurious, beneficial and complete self- exploration of the body.[12]

Create your own feel good plan. And if you are like me, it just has to be fun!

CREATE YOUR OWN PRACTICE

What feels right to me today?

Nourish

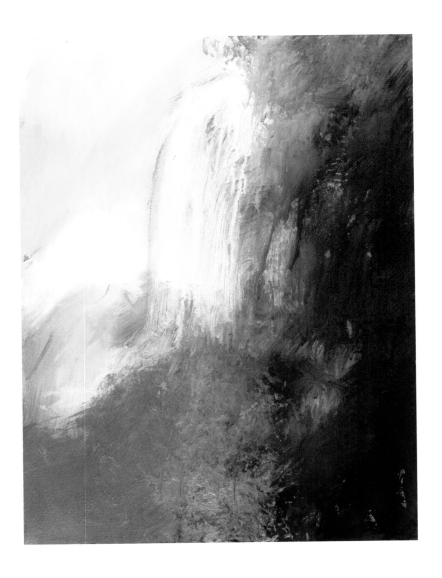

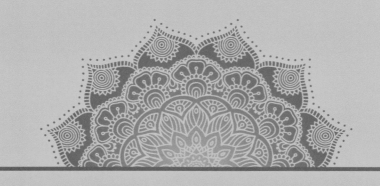

"*Good food enlivens your present and creates your future.*"

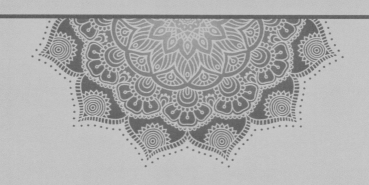

CHAPTER TWO

Nourish

THE ADAGE "YOU ARE WHAT YOU EAT" has had a long and colorful history, and first appeared in English in the 1920's with a quote from nutritionist Victor Lindlahr; "Ninety per cent of the diseases known to man are caused by cheap foodstuffs. You are what you eat."[13] When the quote was popularized in the 1960s, we had the revelation of the relationship between diet and health. Besides movement for basic well-being, the other highly important component is diet, or how you feed yourself. Fast and processed food, pesticides and chemical additives from the food industry are proven to lead to a wide variety of health issues.

Your aliveness and the planet's aliveness are one and the same. Poisons, preservatives, chemicals and unconsciously farmed factory animals are as harmful to the Earth as they are to you. Consuming these products puts an entire segment of the population at risk for obesity, diabetes, neurological disorders and heart conditions as well as dependency on pharmaceuticals for counteracting the conditions they create. This is definitely not self-directed joy of the body! So what is both healthy and sustainable? Eat simply; locally whenever possible. Eat a plant-based diet of fruits and vegetables. If you choose, add organic meats coming from animals that have been fed what they are supposed to eat, such as grass instead of corn for cows. Check the factory conditions of the animals you are consuming. Have they been able to move in their whole life cycle? If not, don't buy or eat them.[14] On a general basis, eliminate all inflammatory-causing foods, such as white flour and sugar. Watch out for GMOs in wheat and grains. Add healthy fats such as nuts, avocado, olive or coconut oil. Many spices and herbs, such as turmeric and oregano add health benefits as well as flavor. Always check labels, as the additives can be shocking.

Eating for maximum health does not really take much extra time or money, especially when compared to the alternative of doctor visits and prescription medications. And it is worth the expansive joy that comes with thoughtful living that makes you feel so vital. It is not necessary to be a vegetarian if that does not work for you. Instead just consider any animal product to be more like a condiment than a main dish. The ultimate diet would be to eat all fresh, preferably organic, with no processed or convenience food. This is not so easy with our busy lives, but with just a little attention, we can get closer to realizing it.

Surprisingly, I found a lot of what works for me when I was changing careers from being a dancer-painter to a full devotion to my Joyous Movement dance programs. This meant that I had to do some financial budgeting during the transition. Because of my creative and complex lifestyle, I require a high energy diet that also produces mental clarity. When I was creating my own unique system, there were so many factors to consider. What would keep me slim, give me loads of energy, maintain lifelong good health, be kind to plants and animals and also taste good? That was a lot to put together. I kept it uncomplicated, buying loads of fresh fruits and vegetables, simple carbohydrates like grains, healthy fats and a bit of fish or chicken. I felt great! Creating a personalized eating program is a path to body connection and is a wonderful self-exploration. Your body is unlike any other, with its own particular likes and dislikes which can change through time. General guidelines are given here, but exactly what works to create your own maximum aliveness will have to be trial and error for you. Ultimately, it is all about just liking the way you feel. When you do your own plan, again be sensitive to how the food makes you feel. After you eat it, are you energetic, slow, sleepy, light, heavy, or satisfied?

Also make sure to eat absolutely whatever you want occasionally when you crave it, but just not in large quantities or all the time. There is joy in that freedom. I find that if I have really overindulged, a day or two of cutting portion size and eating simply will bring me right back. I like a mostly vegetable and protein diet without added sugar, alcohol, or starch for these re-balancing times. Again, this is about feeling good all the time. That is your indicator.

In a nutshell, stay simple, stay fresh, stay local. And by all means, enjoy the pleasure of great food. So for steps one and two, dance and eat plants!

Of course, besides food, nourish yourself in all ways. Sex, swimming, partying, movies, books, trips, walking, hiking, gardening, sailing, puzzles, massage, cloud watching, motor cycle riding—do whatever you love!

STORIES

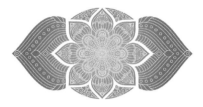

The way you nourish yourself is up to you and the preferences of your body. Food is healing, life-giving and of course, delicious fun.

Jatila van der Veen

For me, being vegetarian is first and foremost a spiritual-ethical-moral decision, and secondly a health-based decision.

I became a vegetarian when I was 23 after having a conversation with one of my housemates. He liked to hunt and fish, and one evening I told him how gross that was. He looked me in the eye and asked if I ate meat. "Yes," I said, "Sometimes." Then he said, "You're a hypocrite if you eat meat but you won't kill it yourself." I was shocked. I looked him in the eye and said, "You're right. From now on I won't eat meat anymore!"

And from that day forward I have not eaten any. At that time I read Diet for a Small Planet, too, which had a profound effect on me in terms of the economics and politics of food. I do eat eggs, but only cruelty-free and antibiotic-free, and I only use beauty products from companies that do not test on animals.

I exercise daily. I stretch and dance every day, and still do splits, high kicks, backbends, and keep up with partners much younger than me. From stage, at least, you can't tell me apart from the

20-and-30-something year olds! I definitely attribute my good health to a healthy lifestyle and vegetarian diet, which started out, first and foremost, as a commitment to non-violence.[15]

Dale Figtree

I always enjoyed tasty food of all kinds although it was never a major focus in my life until I was treated for lymphatic cancer forty years ago. After six months of radiation and chemo, I was told I had exhausted all available treatment, and that there was nothing more the doctors could do for me. That was my wakeup call to shift gears and find another way. I found a Naturopathic Doctor who worked with diet and felt he could do more for me. He put me on a food program of high nutrient foods which I stuck to religiously. At first, the food was my medicine, and I kept it simple. Then I began to work with the foods he suggested in interesting ways. After three years on this intensified food program, and also experiencing many episodes of de-toxing that were naturally stimulated by the super-high food intake, I had a CT scan. The results came back that I was cancer-free!!!!

By that time I developed a deep understanding and appreciation for the healing power of high nutrient food intake and also of the delicious natural flavors in simple healthful foods unhidden by salt and sweeteners. Bit by bit, I created more and more delicious healthful recipes. My food became a joy, not just for me, but also for many others. Just recently I put many of my recipes together in a book called, "Delicious, Nutritious and Simple." That says it all![16]

Aparna Khanolkar

Despite the fact that I was eating healthy and attending college I had no idea of what was brewing in my body. I had just given birth to my son naturally, and simultaneously experienced the loss of my father which was an intense experience for me. I went home to India for a year to heal. After I returned to the U.S. one afternoon a friend noted that I had a lump in my throat. I was shocked by her observation.

I immediately made a doctor's appointment and did all the necessary testing. I was in perpetual anxiety and fear about this. The biopsy revealed that it was a benign complex solid-fluid tumor. The endocrinologist had no idea as to why I got it.

I've always been health conscious so I was puzzled and worried about this new development in my life. I was determined to shrink this tumor in natural ways. I purified my diet, studied the energies of the chakras and how they related to me as a woman.

In retrospect, it was a minor awakening. What was more powerful was the subtle intention. Once the intention was set that I could heal this myself, all doors opened up. In three months, the lump that was hard and poking out of my throat was gone. For seventeen years now, I have been free of any problems. The body is a miraculous organism with its own innate wisdom and intelligence. If we maintain a balance it has powerful capacity to heal and repair itself. It responds to the energetic body faster than anything else. While I know that my multi-faceted approach to holistic healing is what shrank my tumor, it was merely the fixed intention to heal that started the healing process. Even in the midst of this crisis, I did not doubt it. My devotion and commitment to it was so great that healing became inevitable.[17]

SCIENCE

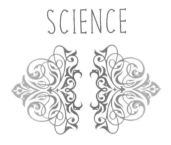

Fueling our bodies is a constant and lifelong activity. Along with our thoughts, food influences the body by providing information-rich biochemical messages to every cell. It can send a positive or negative signal depending on our choices. Food's composition, additives and sources interact with the body at a deep and basic molecular level. The quality of communications from the nutrients that our cells receive to guide them in their basic functioning is an important component in creating vital longevity. Often people do not make the connection between compromised health conditions and their diets.[18]

Nutrients, or the nourishing substances in food such as magnesium, calcium and a variety of vitamins, provide the necessary substances for the body to complete vital processes, like sending nerve impulses and tissue repair. They are essential for growth and the maintenance and development of body functions. Without them our health declines. And when intake does not regularly meet the nutrient needs of cell activity, metabolic processes slow down or even stop.[19] Organic, nutrient-rich foods which don't contain chemical additives do the best job of providing nourishment for our bodies.[20]

From UCLA Professor Fernando Gomez-Pinilla, "Food is like a pharmaceutical compound that affects the brain. This raises the exciting possibility that changes in diet are a viable strategy for enhancing cognitive abilities, protecting the brain from damage and counteracting the effects of aging.[21]

Besides good food for the body's benefit, there is the very important pleasure principle, or enjoyment of the eating experience. High quality visual, auditory and social aspects improve digestion and the assimilation of nutrients. Flavor, aroma, and visual presentation all have health benefits. Thoughtless eating and overindulging can result in negative health consequences such as digestive disorders and obesity. Eating mindfully, on the other hand, encourages proper digestion and can aid in nutrient absorption, promote ideal body weight and help develop a healthy relationship with food.

Thoughtful eating is about bringing awareness and appreciation to the experience of eating. When we eat while under stress or when experiencing busyness or unpleasant emotions, it affects not only what we eat, but how we digest what we eat. When you slow down and pay attention to how and what you eat, you're more likely to make better decisions that will nourish your body. Eating slowly, chewing thoroughly and being in a state of appreciation and gratitude allows full benefit of the food being enjoyed.[22]

By watching portion sizes and eating healthy foods, you can send positive signals to your cells and genes, which increases your chances for a long and vital life. And by taking pleasure in the food you eat and the way you eat it, you will be truly nourished.

PRACTICES

Whenever possible, eat slowly and in good company. Great food is as much nourishment of the soul as it is for the body. Here is a suggested system for you to use as a basis for your own creation. It has worked for me, but please modify it for you own lifestyle and needs. This nutritional program consists of six small meals a day:

Breakfast

One slice gluten free bread with ghee or coconut oil, or a grain like oatmeal.

Choice of Protein: egg, hummus, avocado, sliced turkey, dry cheese such as parmesan.

Vegetables, such as tomato or spinach.

Coconut yogurt with wheat free granola, nuts and fresh fruit such as blueberries.

Snack

One of:

Vegetables and hummus or almond butter.

One fruit selection.

Two ounces of animal protein.

Lunch

Raw vegetable salad such as kale, celery, lettuce, spinach, peppers, jicama with olive oil dressing.

Protein of choice such as shrimp, turkey or chicken breast, salmon, or beans and rice.

Add gluten free pasta or quinoa with olive oil or pesto or a corn tortilla if needing extra energy.

Snack

One of:

Green vegetable drink.

Fruit choice or fruit smoothie.

Dried fruit and almond butter.

Hard boiled egg or other animal protein.

Vegetables and oil dressing of choice.

Dinner

Sautéed or roasted mixed vegetables, any and all of your favorites.

Protein of choice: Beans and rice, turkey breast, chicken, fish, red meat if you occasionally eat it

Snack

Any of the above choices not eaten earlier in the day if still hungry.

Portions

The amount of food is basically determined by stopping just before you get full. This is a practice. Starting with smaller portions than we are usually presented with works well. Experiment with what works for your body.

As a general rule, vegetables are unlimited. Whenever possible, eat organic.

Fruits can be eaten twice a day; grains and starches are eaten once or twice a day. The idea is to keep sugars, even natural, to a minimum.

Protein intake depends on your exercise level, age and gender. In general quantities are approximately four ounces or 120 grams per meal.

I love the sustained energy and flavor of high quality vegetable oils, and eat lots of them on just about everything. Yes, there are good fats! Olive oil, coconut oil, avocados and nut butters are great energy sources and are good for the nervous system. Get creative with spices and combinations to make the simplicity of the food taste great.

Many people love to add juicing to their diets to ensure that they are getting plenty of nutrients. It is also such a pleasure to grow your own herbs or have a small vegetable or tower garden which can be kept even in a small space. I have included some of my favorite recipe and garden growing suggestions in the footnotes.[23]

Again, we all love to celebrate, so remember the pleasure principle. Adhering too strictly to a format, or not allowing yourself to occasionally eat whatever you like, will cause mental anxiety and addictions from either denying yourself or thinking you were "bad." I find that I just make great choices now because I like the way they keep me looking and feeling. I will eat absolutely anything I desire in small amounts and just not all the time. This is not a diet that you can fall off of—it is just everyday eating with a dedication to feeling good!

CREATE YOUR OWN PRACTICE

What feels right to me today?

Release

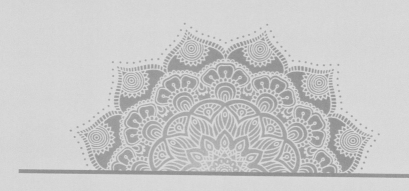

"Letting go and enjoying life now gives the Universe room to work on your behalf."

CHAPTER THREE

Release

THE ACT OF RELEASE or letting go is one of the most important and profound of spiritual practices. Without clearing, there is no access to forward momentum. It is necessary for keeping life fluid and vital. Yet our old pathways of thinking and being are often challenging to release. From letting go of old clothes and possessions to forgiving those who may have hurt us, de-cluttering is one of the most simple and powerful of observances. Have you noticed how many times a day negative beliefs come into mind from the way you have thought before or from past experiences? Beliefs are thoughts we have had over and over again that can color the joy of our presence in the "now." Letting go is said to be the most important spiritual practice. Without it, there is no full existence in the present moment. When we can accept our current conditions in their imperfections and not cement them into the only reality that exists, we can begin to see and feel the next more positive possibilities. It then becomes is easier to let go. Shifting focus from what we are currently thinking about the immediate situation allows its release and then movement into the next more joyful place can occur. Doing this consistently as a way of life means dedication to the desire and belief that feeling good, enjoying life and prospering, is our nature and our right.

The process becomes easier with a clear dedication to a main purpose in life which is to purify our inner awareness so that we can grow. Our consciousness is the lens that is constantly shaping the content of our lives. We can clear or release mental distortions every day by scanning how the thoughts we are perpetually having make us feel. Simply put, if the thought does not make you feel good, it is worth taking at look at it and then re-interpreting and releasing it. New, thoughtful creations can then be put in the empty space. Life at its basis is joyous. With total acceptance of what is, we live in appreciation instead of worry, and appreciation creates beautiful worlds.

There are many methods of identifying and processing limiting beliefs that have been taken on from parents, culture or other authorities.[23] We all have responses to our parents' unconscious behaviors: worry, sadness and anger are the main ones. These reactions are also embedded in our culture, and settle into our brain early on in our lives as automatic responses to situations of pressure. These emotions are signals or clues: we have the ability to transform our experience of them by being aware of them whenever they surface. Just by noticing them, we create the space in our minds to have a different response to them. Identifying thoughts and emotions that don't feel good is the simplest approach to shaping our own experience. I find it is easier and more effective to do this than to continuously reference the past. Looking inside and writing out the embedded viewpoints that I have taken on is my favorite process for becoming familiar with them.

When I am sad, I know it is usually the feeling of lack that is coming up to the surface. This can be a lack of love, safety, resources or worthiness. I can sense its constriction. When this happens, I stop and fully feel and acknowledge the emotion that is present in my heart, mind and body. I breathe into the emotion. When it is fully allowed and accepted, it can be thanked for the insight it offers about my life or unfolding path. With this loving care and attention, a positive opening begins to occur. Then the wealth and love I know to be in the moment reappears. Our lives are created from our inner awareness. In the physical plane constantly occurring situations of learning come through contrast or the appearance of the opposite side of the coin. It is part of how we move through life. There is always some personal insight to be explored under every negative emotion. In this way, we integrate ancient mechanisms of limitations into our expansive lives.

This is a reflective Universe, and circumstances will show up to allow you to see what is inside yourself. Situations that are at odds with your desires are your guideposts, not what is real for you. You have a pattern that you can transform. See what is underneath the fear. Recognize what generates any past habit or compulsive behavior that tries to fill the emptiness. Forgive where it came from. Feel the emotions and then move through them. There is great joy in these discoveries and a deepening relationship to the self that gives life a stability that is fun. Don't fear it – welcome it! Life is endlessly entertaining when approached this way. As we continue more with these practices, having strength and confidence becomes a grounded way of life.

STORIES

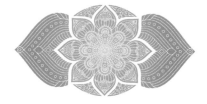

Release and the Body

Often physical symptoms such as colds or injuries are calls from the inner self through the body to slow down and take notice of what is going on at a deeper level. The causation of current circumstances can be revealed, related to, and a new happier place can be created. I recently had a cold and cough that would not go away and there was no real reason for my immune system to be compromised. With the help of talking to a close girl friend and my sister along with a few nights of resting, I got the message that the cold was about unconscious congestion from the past. In order to move forward in my life's mission of being joyous and celebrating with others, I noticed what was making me unhappy. It was limiting feelings about my capability to expand into a larger world of relationship as an artist through a thriving business. Since this growth is my deepest and most heartfelt desire, I could then immediately refocus on what a pleasure it is going to be to meet new people and move forward into a richer more expansive life. We all consistently make up our stories and can rewrite and choose any possibility! The very act of writing it all out was helpful, and I use this technique when other areas such as relationship fears come up. The blockage was cleared and I was back to vibrant health and feeling deserving of all of it. The old habit can occasionally re-appear, so keep refocusing on the new desired reality and the journey of your next step appearing will be delicious.

Roxy Angel Superstar
The power of forgiveness

I have always been told by the home and hearth crew (my family, clergy etc.) that if I held on to my bitterness and rage and did not forgive and turn the other cheek, (especially on some people like family members) I would never know a day of peace. All that input did was make my beef simmer in quiet and never offered me the way out of the hellishness of not forgiving.

I was tired of carrying around a lifetime of hatred toward my family and baby daddy. How corrosive and bitter it felt to be holding onto that pain. Thankfully I was taking a class at a center I was attending to help me stop the self pity and disappointment that was blocking the joy in life for me. My teacher said "Girl, I know what your solution is for all your problems. If you do this you are going to be so free." I answered, "Sign me up" because I was feeling anything but free.

So this righteous Reverend says "You need to do the Seven times Seventy forgiveness exercise. I want you to write down seventy times a day for seven days straight, 'I love you Daddy and I forgive you." I was in such pain that the first day I wrote it, I felt like I was in child birth.

I was forgiving a man who didn't want to see me, a man who I blamed for every unhappiness and terror of my childhood. It took five days for me to start surrendering to the forgiveness process. By day six, I wrote that phrase seventy times again and to my utter surprise, I felt lighter and actually had zero tears.

By day seven, I felt nothing! In fact, I felt what I was writing was utterly true. I knew that it was exactly what the doctor ordered and was so profound for healing my feelings so much. I felt cleansed out and lighter in mind and heart than I had ever felt before.

Two weeks later, my Gramma telephoned me and said "Your father is dying and you don't have time to waste, get here now." Are you kidding? How is this coming up now? I just forgave him! I stood at my father's death bed holding his hand.

I freely expressed my feelings, telling him that I hadn't felt he had loved me ever. He was there, if unable to speak, holding on to my hand for dear life, tears streaming behind his closed eyes. Telling me in no words just how sorry he was, how much he appreciated me and our family being with him in this moment.

My father died in peace two days later. I attended his funeral and I became less broken.

I never imagined how powerful forgiveness could ever be. I felt whole, and closer to my family than ever had before. Forgiveness is the only way I grew up and became a human. Grace moves in mysterious ways; never bypass the opportunity to forgive.[24]

Deanna Cohen
The importance of de-cluttering

Good Feng Shui is the healthy and unobstructed flow of energy in the environment, affecting your health, livelihood, relationships and opportunities positively. As a Feng Shui Consultant, when I walk into a living space and see that it is unorganized and cluttered, I know that there is something out of balance in the person's life, and that the clutter and disarray is contributing to that imbalance. Clutter is stagnant, congested, unprocessed and depressed energy that effectively drains your energy, to the point of eventually becoming debilitating. It also negatively impacts, or completely blocks the flow of energy in the events of your life. You can go along for quite some time thinking that clutter has nothing to do with why life is tiring and full of obstacles, but the radical transformation that is experienced once the clutter is gone, is undeniable. The outside world reflects it by suddenly bringing you the opportunities you desire and the new found energy to accomplish them by.

In order to get a feel for the clutter in your environment, start by looking at each room, cupboard, closet, desk top objectively, paying close attention to the feeling you have when you look at what is in front of you. Is it overwhelming? Do you feel agitated and confused? This is what is affecting you subconsciously every time you walk into the room, open your cupboard or closet, or sit down at your desk. De-cluttering becomes very exciting once you realize this.

It can at times be challenging to de-clutter on your own, given the attachment you may feel to certain things, such as clothing you think one day you will wear, or a broken appliance you've been hoping to fix but haven't, or magazines and newspapers that aren't being read because they are no longer relevant or are lost under a bunch of other stuff.

Sometimes it helps to employ someone to walk you through the process, someone who doesn't have the same attachment to your clutter as you do and can see things with fresh eyes. Keep in mind, de-cluttering can be a very emotional process as things get stirred up and you get out of your comfort zone. The process however will reveal how your disorder has been holding you back, but in the end you will feel exhilarated because you are creating fresh new pathways for vibrant energy to flow into your home, allowing you to live your life more fully.[25]

SCIENCE

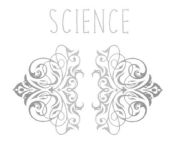

The release of old or unwanted pathways of thought is liberation into life. Consider the possibility that resistance to the new and keeping things as they are, cause blockages that manifest physically in the body and brain. Our systems were meant to keep fresh and open to exploring. We can learn at any age and keep our minds and neurons (electrical brain cells that transmit information to our bodies) flexible. With elasticity of mind and heart, our re-created selves expand in sync with the universe that we are part of.

The brain has a range of electronic signals, somewhat like a scale of musical notes. They are called brainwaves and are a spectrum of our consciousness that allows us to either tie our shoes or go into deep creativity. They change according to what we are doing or feeling.[26]

Alpha brain waves contain the power of intuition and being in the now. They are the gateway to the subconscious mind and lie at the base of conscious awareness. Old patterns can be accessed and cleared in the relaxed Alpha state. The mind's most deep-seated programs are at Theta and this is where we experience vivid visualizations, great inspiration, profound creativity and exceptional insight. It is said that a sense of deep spiritual connection and unity with the universe can be experienced at Theta.[27]

It is at the Alpha-Theta border, where the optimal range for visualization, mind programming and using the creative power of your mind begins. It's the mental state in which you can consciously create your reality. At this frequency, you are conscious of your surroundings, however your body is in deep relaxation. Forgiveness creates the Alpha-Theta brain waves of higher consciousness. Even just pretending to forgive allows the mind to experience this state and create a shift.[28]

But the brain is not the sole driver of our experience that we once thought it was. The brain and the heart are linked. Newest research reveals that the heart has a much bigger and more powerfully radiant electro-magnetic field. Our brain gets its signals from the heart which tells the brain what to communicate to the body. Most important is the power of feeling, and the connection between thought, emotion and feeling. This is how we manifest our worlds as feelings enliven or speak to the blueprints of our desires.[29]

Scientists now know that all matter is interconnected. It is continuous vibration. The energy of our large heart fields also interconnects with everyone we are in contact with. How open is your heart? What are you feeding the world each day with your thoughts? Imagine a collective expansion of heart-based living. That is the possibility for increased global coherence and continuous peace.[30]

Free any boundaries on the heart that mind habits may have generated. De-clutter external environments, as well as the mind and emotions.[31] With release, room is made for the receptive process of allowing. Breathe, let go and refresh.

PRACTICES

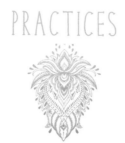

I have included some of my favorite practices for release or letting go of unwanted, no longer valid or necessary energy of the past so that new and fresh desires have room to appear. Life is constantly transitional and therefore requires perpetual fluidity with circumstances, thoughts and even your dreams.

1. Get rid of all that old stuff that is cluttering up your physical environment! I am always astounded at the clarity and release of energy that happens when I get rid of clothes, papers, or anything with dead energy that is not useful in the present. This can be done a little at a time, or regularly every month. I personally clear my physical environment whenever I feel a blockage or obstacle, which can often happen. Sometimes, the congestion is in my office, sometimes in my garden and often in my closet.

2. Allow some time every day, perhaps even just 10 minutes, to feel what is going on with you. Stuck feelings can be identified by the fact that something does not feel good; it can even be a discomfort in your body. Open up to the fear, sit with it, breathe and allow it. Everything hidden comes out and this easy process brings it to light in a healthy, loving way.

Once the thoughts and emotions are identified, it is possible to detach from negative concepts of self in order to create the future in the now and release the limitations of the past. What would you prefer to be thinking? If limiting thoughts return, they are easier to just identify and not be listened to or made real.

These times with yourself are also a place of devotion. Forgive yourself often, which is a practice in being completely kind and accepting. Be with what is and love. Everything comes from being in the moment and everything is available in the present moment.

3. Hold yourself as beautiful and complete as you are now, instead of thinking something has to be fixed. Release perfectionism. Besides not being fun, it does not allow for the uncertainty and openness of creative process that can lead you on an expansive adventure elsewhere. Self-love is a reflection of divine love. Any separation from this is a product of the mind. We are innately completely valuable, worthy and loved.

4. Practice acceptance of others, even though you may not agree with them in any way. There are always going to be vast differences and varieties of viewpoints. It is not necessary to engage intimately with those who are not compatible with your beliefs, but there will be a lot less mental clutter and personal unhappiness to clear with less judgment of others. It is okay release the people in your life that don't make you happy or add to it in some positive way. This is learning to be kinder to and more accepting of yourself and your preferences.

5. Live in appreciation instead of worry. Find things in your life to appreciate all day long. The money you have, the air, the running water, everything you have and are! Feeling good

now equals always the presence of the eternal. It is the end of the endless chase to be something else or be somewhere else. Focus more on what is going right, and more of what is going right will occur. This is the practice of living the fullness of the moment of what is.

6. Check any discomfort or negative emotions regularly. Where are they coming from and what do they want to tell you?

7. It is a reflective Universe. Be aware that you can attract those who will mirror or show you your wounded or separated self. It is a special gift, so that you can see more clearly and be freer and filled with light. There becomes a constant refinement of what you attract into your experience.

8. Escape the prison of self-limitation including that of quantifying numbers, such as age or weight.

9. Praise yourself often as a reflection of the wonder and beauty of being alive. You are made of the earth and the stars.

10. Use a forgiveness process if needed.

Liberating Forgiveness Process:
Reverend Maryum Morse, Santa Barbara

Forgiveness creates the alpha/theta brain waves of higher consciousness. Even just pretending to forgive will allow you to feel that state and will shift you. Allow the dark to come up to clear the energy.

1. Say a prayer, opening to receive and that higher wisdom is assisting.

2. Choose the person you would like to forgive. Do one person at a time.

3. What emotion are you feeling? Anger, sadness, hatred?

4. Where are you feeling it in your body?

5. What color is it?

6. Write down the entire list of everything you can think of that you feel this person has done to you, whatever you need to forgive them for. Neglect, abuse, infidelity, whatever it is.

7. Say " I need to forgive you for_____."

8. Then say the person's name and say: I would have preferred that you_____ me. But you didn't do that and you never will do that so I have no choice but to cancel that expectation of you.

9. Get it out of your body by crossing your arms in front of your chest and then opening them in a clearing motion. Do this out loud, yell if it pleases you and use as much emotion as is coming out of you.

10. Do this process for each item on your list.

11. Say to them: I forgive you. If you can't do that, say God or any other term you like to use for this such as Spirit, Universe, or Higher Self forgives you.

12. Say "I wish you well" (meaning you wish their spirit well).

13. Say "I send you Divine love and I take my power back NOW." Get physical when you do this.

What are you feeling now in that place where it resided in your body? What color is it now?[32] Forgive yourself often. You are complete!

Release/Transition Using Shrines

Times of transition are some of the most difficult in the letting go process, and this is because they are so uncomfortable. The transition can be in a relationship (such as divorce or separation), in finances or career (job loss or change), or in moving locations. The life- style changes they provoke require release of old habits and familiar ways of being. It takes courage to leap off, a steadfastness and deep belief that all is working out.

Clear space is required, almost like a cleansing or a fast, so that a detoxification of the past occurs. It is then possible to live in the emptiness until the new emerges. We are just not culturally trained for appreciating empty space. It is a death of sorts, which also turns into the womb of pure possibility. After the discomfort is ridden through, the benefit, or the art that is made from the process is a new sense of faith and trust in life. Our lives are refined and now lived at a higher level. I have found the ancient power of ritual or sequence of acts to be very effective in both processing and releasing feelings. A shrine is an enclosed space that contains internal life and this process combines the two together. This particular ritual uses a combination of shrines; one for clearing and one for the peace of empty space. A third can then be used for creating new beginnings. Here is my ritual for the discomfort of transition:

Choose or create a Purification shrine, and sit comfortably in front of it, eyes closed. Breathe in and out evenly, realizing that life is in constant flux, forever dying, casting off form, and then renewing itself with fresh experience. Stay until you are comfortable with the evenness of your breath. Allow feelings to surface. Take as long as you like. Write down the feelings. Move your body with them. Then burn the paper or put it in the release shrine for purification. Sit with the not knowing saying "I release the past. I trust in life and I am set free. I am open to new experience and new possibilities, and I embrace their freshness. New life, show me the way!" Then focus on the empty Peace shrine and breathe and savor the spaciousness and light that is filling your body. Light a candle. Whenever you become ready to allow it to come in, choose a creation ritual for the fresh reality of choice, open to a new now and fresh future. The Universe is conspiring to give us a life which is unencumbered by history. It is wide open and all we have to do is remember everything is coming to fruition. Now be totally in your life to love it and share it in joy.[33]

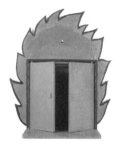

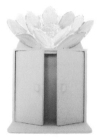
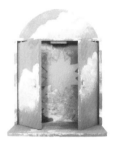

Purification   *Peace*   *Creation*

CREATE YOUR OWN PRACTICE

What feels right to me today?

Give

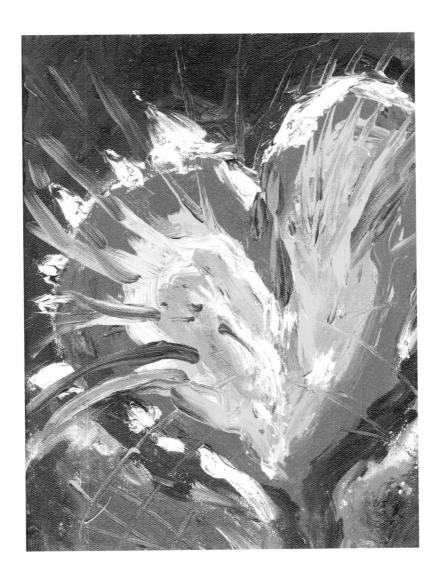

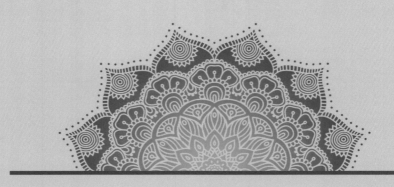

"Opening your heart to others is the surest way to expand your own capacity to receive love and is the biggest gift you can give to yourself."

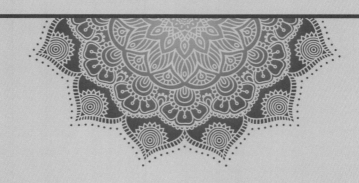

CHAPTER FOUR

Give

EXPANDING THE BOUNDARIES OF YOUR HEART and expressing kindness is a sure fire way to light up your own cells. I have experienced this time and time again with seniors of limited physical and mental capabilities. Just by being with them, I begin to have a non-judgmental experience through music and movement. We all light up. The beauty of their encased spirits is liberated, and I am filled with the radiance of life as well.

Service is a kind of purification. It is in its essence connecting to the light and more uplifting aspects of life. The trick is to give without seeing a need or deficit in the person or group. Focusing on any condition just amplifies it. Instead, it is about relating to the wholeness or glow of the life energy that is present regardless of the form.

Giving has taught me much about relating to the essence of what is in front of me instead of its physical illusion. I believe that our highest value as humans is compassion. This means that I see myself in you. That view not only enlarges your being, but also changes the planet and is one of the most powerful and innovative practices for world transformation. It can be as simple as a smile. Give a few every day, and that smile will most likely come back to you. Everyone responds to this pure heart energy. Practicing being non-judgmental is so fulfilling and can lead to some of the most profound connections with people who do not look like who they really are inside. Tolerance for the Earth's variety is a far-reaching practice. Greet everyone with love and they will reflect it back to you. This is deep, spiritual food and it will rejuvenate you daily.

I learned this simple practice of opening up boundaries and eliminating separation in a most unexpected way. My unique way to serve is throwing dance parties. I know this because nothing makes me happier than having great music and a community of people who are experiencing joy together. While performing dinner shows at Middle Eastern Restaurants for much of my life, I quickly learned that it was the shish kebab or me! I performed at a large restaurant in Santa Barbara through much of the 1970s and 1980s which often had 200 people in the round each night. I quickly realized that if I opened my heart energy and gave a smile and made eye contact with as many as possible, I could unite the energy of the room in joy and well-being. I actually had control of the vibration of the room.

This led to the development of Joyous Movement, my fun dance fitness programs for every body, which have helped many people of every age, ability and condition to find their own joy through dance celebration. These techniques are the same as those that are taught to all Joyous Movement instructors. They have biochemical reactions, as well as the simple and most profound goal of living in enjoyment and happiness, which is our essential nature.

Find a way to serve that is unique to your being. Explore where you love to give. We are unlimited beings with an endless capacity for love.

STORIES

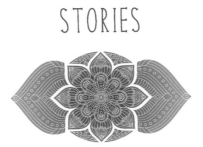

Balanced loving interaction or service without looking for a result or reward has been a great source of happiness and rejuvenation for me. Here are stories from a couple of world servers:

Janet Reineck

In my life, I've been a dancer, anthropologist, and humanitarian aid worker. In 2010, I set out to bring these parts of my life together and started a nonprofit, "World Dance for Humanity." Our dance classes offer a chance for women to connect with each other, and with the world, while helping people in need. All the proceeds go to our work in Rwanda, where we are helping Genocide survivors lift themselves out of poverty and rebuild their lives. We have created a compassionate community of dancers here at home, and a passionate partnership with people on the other side of the planet.

This quote from Anne Frank sums up my feeling about service: "How wonderful it is that nobody need wait a single moment before starting to improve the world."

Working for 8 years in Kosovo (former Yugoslavia), and 4 years in Rwanda, taught me what it's like for people all over the world who live and die in hardship and hopelessness. I learned from these experiences that service is everything: it's what life is about. I wake up every day astounded that I have a bed to sleep in, running water and food to eat. I jump out of bed, propelled by a desire to make something happen that will ease the suffering that is all around us. My motto is: "Do good, and disappear."[34]

Anaiya Mussolini

The light inside me shines brightest when globally advocating for orphans and empowering women through dance. Deep inside, I always knew being a children's advocate was my calling. When I decided to fully pursue this path, the world created serendipitous ways to entertain my other true passion of dance. That is the gift in giving; you receive far more in return than you would ever imagine. Transformation begins. When following your dreams, the world creates opportunities within so many other dimensions of your life: to provide support, but only if you possess the courage to pursue what truly lies in your heart.

On one of my trips to volunteer at orphanages I led multiple belly dancing empowerment workshops helping the Dhapasi women, a lower cast group of marginalized women in Nepal. A center there offers educational life training and other beneficial opportunities to these disenfranchised women. They were so grateful to participate in these dance workshops, but it was I who was overcome with gratitude. For when you share a part of yourself (the most sacred truest part) to people in need, that is rasa - the essence of art. Feeling blessed to be part of these women's lives and help them through pain, just as people helped me when I so needed it in the past. And what fun way to challenge the dark side, letting it out thought the light of dance. When you give, the world gives to you.[35]

SCIENCE

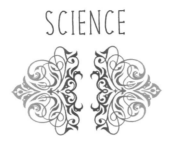

There are many physiological as well as psychological benefits to giving or being of service. Beyond helping others, we are helping ourselves.

Giving lowers blood pressure, decreases depression and offers longer life and greater happiness. Biologically, it can create a warm glowing feeling and activate regions in the brain associated with pleasure, connection and trust.

Generosity increases self-esteem and self-love, leading to more positive emotions which affect the body's biochemistry. There is evidence that during gift-giving behaviors, feel good chemicals in our brains such as serotonin (a mood mediating chemical), dopamine (a feel good chemical) and oxytocin (a bonding and compassion chemical) are secreted.

Supportive interaction with others also helps people recover from coronary related events such as heart attacks and cardiac arrests. It has been found that giving stimulates the reward center in the brain, releasing endorphins and creating what is known as the supporter's Helper's High. Using the heart center decreases the chances of heart disease.[36]

Our amazing human hearts pump life-giving oxygenated and nutrient-rich blood throughout our bodies on a precise schedule. Now researchers are learning that this marvelous machine, the size of a fist and weighing on average less than 10 ounces, also possesses a level of intelligence which they are only beginning to understand. Evidence shows that the heart also plays a greater role in our mental, emotional and physical processes than previously thought.

Research from the Heart Math Institute Director, Rollin McCraty, says that the heart is a sensory organ and acts as a sophisticated information encoding and processing center that enables it to learn, remember and make independent functional decisions.

The heart, like the brain, generates a powerful electromagnetic field, actually the largest in the body, almost 60 times greater than that of brain waves. Studies also show that this powerful electromagnetic field can be detected and measured several feet away from a person's body. When people touch or are in proximity, a transference of the electromagnetic energy produced by the heart occurs. Through the use of tools and technologies that foster positive emotions and mind-body coherence, individuals can effectively initiate a re-patterning process. Habitual emotional patterns that underlie stress are replaced with newer healthier ones. This establishes increased emotional stability, mental acuity and physiological efficiency as a new familiar baseline or norm.[37]

Positive emotions such as appreciation, caring, compassion and gratitude set up a connection between our hearts and mind.[38] There is a relationship between positive emotions, expressed love and healthy hearts and bodies. So express yourself!

PRACTICES

An easy place to begin giving is to expand small gestures of kindness in some way every day, even if it is just one smile to someone you don't know. Opportunities for simple acts like allowing a car to go in front of you in traffic or having an encouraging conversation are constantly available. These exchanges enlarge the spirit and just feel good.

Find a place to give that stretches your boundaries and yet is something that is uniquely you. This is another opportunity for self-exploration. What are your interests? Are they cooking, traveling, flower arranging, horseback riding, accounting, assisting the elderly? There are places you can find to serve with whatever it is that you enjoy.

At the most basic level, what you are giving is who you essentially are and what you are radiating is the point around which the experience of everyone you interact with unfolds. What is foremost is the desire to feel more expression and unconditional love in yourself first. These qualities are what are infectious and open others up. Express and share the joy of life.

Over my long history of both teaching dance and being an entertainer, I have discovered many effective methods of connecting with an individual, group or audience to create a unified, open, safe and expressive space for everyone. Some of these techniques are subtle and internal, while others are glittery and worn on the outside. It is a non-verbal felt communication, the unspoken language of the heart and the body. Here are a few simple practices to free your own radiance:

Generate a positive feeling. Think of something pleasant like a pet or the smiles of children, whatever lights you up. Let it infuse your body and being. Stretch up and breathe and then sparkle through the door to whatever room you enter!

Go on a binge of appreciating all you have that allows you to give. Health, running hot water, transportation, cool outfits and a heart that desires to expand are a few of mine, what are yours?

Hold the hands of a friend, gaze in their eyes and give them a look of love. This works wonders on any of the elderly I see regularly. You can use this look with anyone, without any bodily contact. Let the smile you get back radiate through your entire body.

The best exercise for releasing internal barriers to sharing your unique radiance is to consistently practice all these techniques. Everyone will have their own style and capacity for non-judgmental love and compassion for others. There are deeper benefits to this as well. The release of all loving energies creates an internal purification. I have noticed more self confidence, better health and the joy of more self-love.

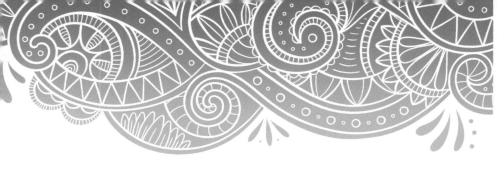

CREATE YOUR OWN PRACTICE

What feels right to me today?

Create

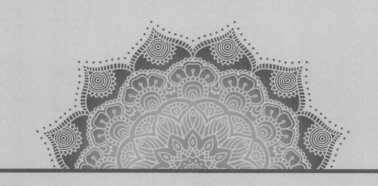

"*Live daily on the edge of your own growth.*"

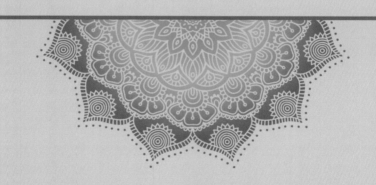

CHAPTER FIVE

Create

A FAVORABLE RELATIONSHIP TO THE UNKNOWN is crucial to happiness. We live in a world of infinite possibilities, and the ability to access them is one of the gifts of being human. Creative thinking puts you in a deep and pleasurable relationship with the current moment. There are no mistakes, anything can happen. Improvisation keeps the neural pathways fresh and open, which is crucial to lifelong brain fitness. Most importantly, new ideas produce comfort with the constant expansion that is one of the basic qualities of life itself. The ultimate creation is the choices we make to craft our own lives and become who we have imagined.

We are all in flux, works in progress. Of course, there is disorder or chaos and places of discomfort, but from my experience, with perseverance the art that is inherent in any situation always comes to pass. Perfection is a highly overrated concept in our culture as it denies the liberating permutations of creative process. Are you brave enough to live with this? The choice is always yours, "Do I want that or not?" Flow, deep enjoyment and greater peace then become the fabric of life. When I teach art, especially to children, I always say "There are no mistakes in art." They are completely astounded that a reality exists where this is possible. I then add, "Life is like that as well." Every path leads you somewhere, and the decision to make the next turn is yours. An enjoyed journey leads to a happy destination.

Humans are powerful deliberate creators, the only species that can alter and choose their own future. This is much like making a work of art. The inspiration or idea comes from connecting to a Universal place. Then the design emerges. And finally its materialization happens by allowing the manifestation come through.

Creating the life of your dreams is a similar three part process. First, take the time to get an awareness of what you most want in your life; what you would like it to look like. This is the blueprint for reality or the idea. Next, is to know that the answer is always "Yes". You do have the power to have and to create whatever you desire. We live in a very generous Universe! Everything gets made twice, once in the imagination and then in physical reality. This is the ancient axiom, "as above, so below". It becomes real the moment that the thought happens. The last step is to be a co-operative component in your desires coming to fruition by being in a relaxed state that allows them to unfold. This is often the most challenging part, as we are culturally trained to do and control. Making art is a great way to learn this creative process of allowing or being receptive, which is a newer, more feminine approach. I have found that the minute I begin trying to completely control the outcome of a medium such as paint, the magic is gone. So let go and let it come through. Say: "I am a co-operative component of my desire. I believe in what I want and that I already have it."

Play often. Follow the fun! Do what feels fresh and good as a pervasive approach to life. Creating something keeps you on the cutting edge of becoming. It is great to not know. Keeping the neural pathways open can add much enjoyment to life, as solutions will come in to solve routine challenges. Do something new every day. This can be as simple as taking a new route to work. I am a big advocate of including art of any type that pleases you in your life as a pleasurable path to inner knowing and revealing. If you are human, you are creative. And yes, anyone can do it! Having taught autistic children, women at risk, stressed out executives, war trauma victims and many regular folk, I have personally witnessed that everyone is an artist with something unique to express. A sense of stability about welcoming the unknown feels both alive and peaceful at the same time.

STORIES

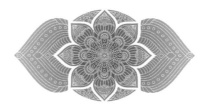

I am constantly taught by the creative process. I know that I will always get to the destination, and that the road to the completed art work or design of any kind is an unknown adventure. I have an entry area in my garden that cannot grow grass because of all the traffic. I saw a gravel path at a friend's house and decided to try that as a solution and bought some lovely small stones. When I put them down, this spray of white rocks felt intrusive and uncomfortable visually. Then I let go and got into that delicious process. Arranging and adding beach rocks, glass gems and sea glass made it more suitable to my aesthetic and inner world and I loved it. By continuously feeling, I got to know my inner authentic self.

Not long after this I had some discomfort or challenges with possibilities that came in for fulfilling my largest intentions. This was at a time in my life around the selection of business collaborators for bringing my life's work to the world. No one had worked out, those who showed up were not a fit. I know that this is one of the places of my greatest internal growth so I paid attention. It threw me for a spin momentarily until I found a number of ways to realign. The first one was to not focus on the pain of the not fitting but gratitude that I had energetic possibilities that I drew to myself. It was like laying down that first layer of gravel. I remembered that life is a fluid process of inner growth. Who I am becoming is the art that is being revealed.

I became open to the next step or set of possibilities to arrive, and it was like adding the jewels to the stones. I learned what would work better for me, a refinement and progression of choices. With this approach, I could welcome all the phases instead of reacting negatively and could receive the riches of enjoying the journey.

Shannon Jaffe
Art Instructor to 500 children at
Monroe Elementary, Santa Barbara, CA

It has been my experience that students thrive during art making. They learn to trust themselves and others. I have had several high school age teens come to art without the willingness to draw or share their work. After 3 months, I noticed that they opened up their sketchbooks, drew a self-portrait and trusted their environment enough to share in a community mural.

Children learn to take risks and make mistakes. Elementary age students often come to art with the fear of making a wrong choice. After learning to trust their surroundings in the art room, they become confident enough to try something new and create with their imagination. Eventually, they even lose the restriction that an adult has to approve their expressions.

Working together becomes part of the freedom and fun. Students who claim to "hate" art end up enjoying working with their friends on collaborative projects like murals. They learn that they can accomplish meaningful pieces that are recognized by the community, while boosting their self esteem.

Art making teaches life skills through encouraging meditative states that allow students of all ages to experience how to get to that place, "the zone." I watch pre-school age children and kindergarteners relax when they come into the art room. They understand that the expectation is there for them to create without an end result or product and this releases anxiety and stress. They are given room to blossom.[39]

Seyburn Zorthian

Painting has been an intense lifetime exploration for me. Creativity can arise from ideas -sometimes generated to solve a problem - or from feelings, which are induced by our perceptions of the world, nature, other beings and ourselves. It is deeply fulfilling to bring these concepts into being through the creative process. This requires being open to the unknown. I can't cling to preconceived standards of what is good or bad work, because that gets in the way of my creative expression. I have to be willing to let something emerge and suspend my impulse to judge while I allow the work to develop.

The painting starts with the first impression, a color wash or an expressive line, and the rest of the process intuitively follows as a cumulative series of responses like an improvisation in music or dance. As in music and dance, there are self-imposed structures like the size or media used that create a space where you have freedom to explore what is actually important. That's where the openness comes in. To me, cultivating that necessary sense of openness is a big part of being an artist.[40]

SCIENCE

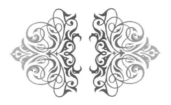

Creative activities and thinking are restorative. Participating in them increases well-being by replacing negative emotions and conditions with positive ones. We become trained in the qualities of flow and spontaneity. There is true power in the personal decision making they require. On a spiritual level, life is drawn through us. These uplifted states also have a profound effect on our health and produce real physical changes in the body. The practiced connections develop our own authority to heal ourselves.[41] Activities such as writing can actually impact our cells and improve the immune system. A creative project is an opportunity to ignore incoming signals of media and information that continuously bombard us and generate our very own authentic outward signals. Benefits come because it FEELS good.[42]

For brain health, the axiom is use it, or lose it. The brain is very malleable and has a great capacity to change. Having many neural pathways to information is more beneficial than having one well worn route. A greater amount of neural synapses or connections creates greater possibilities for accessing information. With only one neural pathway connecting to stored information, we can become blocked. Some memory loss can be a natural process, especially if the mind is not kept active. Participating in mentally engaging activities produces more new neural paths. The brain constantly rewires itself depending on use, and more is better. But if it isn't used, it won't make any more. Keep the paths active and create new ones. The opposite of this is taking the same old well-worn mind path over and over again, with habitual patterns of thinking and living our lives. More approaches allow more fluidity and unique expression.[43]

The use of the imagination to create new habits is stimulating and life-giving. A redundant set of practiced behaviors or reactions is like a software program that runs automatically. It keeps repeating as stimulus pushes the same button and we are never truly present. Many people wait for a crisis or trauma to stimulate change and to notice what they are doing and thinking unconsciously. Then they can see and no longer be identified with that repetitive program. But this awareness can come without the need for devastating and shocking experiences. You can create change through choice and a devotion to the joy of life. Change can happen through inspiration and a desire to live your very own vision of the future.

There is a neurology (science of the nervous system) to creativity and transformation. Our frontal lobe is the center or director of the brain. When it is stimulated with a question or a creative idea, it links all parts of the brain cohesively to access information. A new level of understanding is created from this synthesis and we have a vision. Then there is a process to bring it to life. You can be newly defined by your vision by releasing what you know you don't want and re-visiting and focusing on what you do want. The brain is pruning and sprouting neurologically. When the moment occurs that this new identity is desired more than living the old emotions, our systems relax. The mind and body link electro-magnetically with the design. With self-love and self-respect, the new vision is allowed to unfold and be received. If attention of the conscious mind is kept on the vision, the subconscious will bring it to pass. It is not possible to be a victim if you are creating, as you are emulating your unlimited or divine self. Creativity connects you with this expansive intelligence.

Live and believe your project or dream, even though you can't see it yet. With emotion, love your vision so much that your body and mind accept it as true that you are already living that future. The brain and body will make biological and quantum changes. Combining heart and mind broadcasts this new signature. All possibilities exist in the present moment, so re-visit and align with your positive vision of the future and allow it to come to you. It is yours.[44]

PRACTICES

There are many ways to be creative and form innovating new mind pathways. It is the process of allowing visions to come to life. You have the ability to feel your way to a manifestation of original design. This can be anything that births something which is uniquely an expression of you; as simple as a change in a recipe or as complex as the design of a new car engine. Solution-generated thinking for any of life's varied challenges becomes natural, part of the flow of life. Living in continuous expansion is a reflection of life's essential nature and is constantly rejuvenating. It is play!

One of everyone's most important creations of all is the content of the story of our lives. How it is told it is completely individual. It can be continuously revised to its most positive aspects; it becomes the blueprint for what happens. You are creating all the time, so watch your words. Words are powerful and make worlds come into being. I am often astounded at all the negative talk I hear, especially about people's bodies. Through words, we can totally shift our attitudes and our resolve to create the reality we most desire for ourselves.

Set aside some time for this directive. The easiest way to begin is to become quiet and first ask often, "What would I love?" This can be a very profound process. Journaling, vision boards and dreamtime in a receptive state can be used. Yes, you can have it! Remember, the world is your playground, imagine big.

1. What would the life you would love to have look like?

2. Know that you can have it; it is possible.

3. Clear old beliefs if necessary or if you are feeling conflict about your worthiness to have it.

4. Be open to receive and allow it to unfold.

5. Feel having it in the now and let go. Connect to your vision with the emotions.

6. Take divinely guided or inspired actions.

7. Offer gratitude. It is the journey of getting there that is all the fun!

Your life or source energy becomes a match to the design and you become a part of the point of attraction which brings to you the ideas, circumstances and individuals that will fulfill your desires. It is joyful to witness our co-creative capacity and see all the synchronistic and miraculous components emerge. Events unfold that you will see as opportunities that you would not have recognized before you had the connection to your vision. You will be in the right place at the right time. Be in a relaxed understanding that everything you imagined is coming into full fruition. Dream big and enjoy each step of its unfolding.

Make sure that attention to your existing situations don't become more real to you than your vision – they are only temporary. Current conditions are not as real as your new story.

Review your dream story without judgment. Just know the beauty of your desire to expand and that it is the nature and law of reality for it to be fulfilled.

Find the humor in most situations and look for a positive interpretation. Think outside the box. Listen and connect to divine sources of inspiration. Be in a state of flow. We tend to perceive conditions as fixed, but everything in life is flexible in the moment. The art is in shifting the focus of the mind from current results to the possibilities that we desire. The alchemy is in looking at and accepting situations that appear as disparities or blockages to your imagined life. Instead, see them as choices, or guideposts that are showing you your way by revealing what you don't want, so that you can further refine what you do want. They then become a light for you, rather than a dark dead-weight.

Develop the habit of opening the mind daily. Take five minutes with your morning cup to dream, appreciate and expand. Have some fun visioning - as big as you can. We are taught to shut down with age and that decline is inevitable. I believe the opposite is true. It is as easy to cultivate life. And it so much more fun!

CREATE YOUR OWN PRACTICE

What feels right to me today?

Join

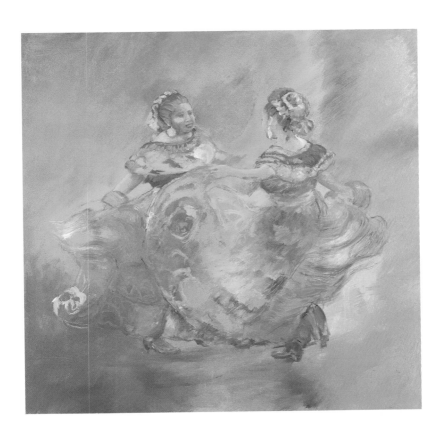

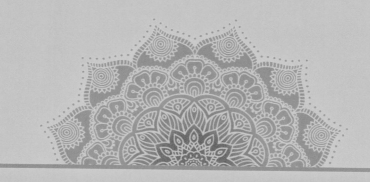

"Connecting with others in delight
expands the boundaries of self."

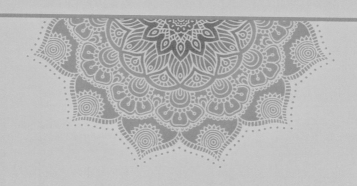

CHAPTER SIX

Join

HUMANS ARE A COMBINATION OF socially interdependent beings and the individual creators of their own world. We are innately and biologically wired as a tribe or social group and studies show that those with no social contact live shorter, sadder lives. Our bodies are co-operative components of trillions of cells that constantly communicate. On a molecular level, we are all interconnected. Collaboration, along with compassion, are the two most important components for building a new sustainable life on our planet. Like our cells and bodies, in groups or co-operative communities, we can take care of each other and provide a sense of belonging to the whole. The welfare of one individual component increases the well-being of all.

The benefits of socializing are many. It can relieve the stress and anxiety of feeling all alone, increase mental functioning through the sharing of ideas and provide all types of support. It fosters an understanding of others and increases self-confidence through interacting. Science is proving that unifying with others is crucial to mental and physical health. And of course, getting together provides what I consider to be the greatest curative which is the opportunity to celebrate! Whether holding hands with a group of individuals with memory loss issues or participating in a full blown dance theater party, I notice the deep joy that is produced from creating connection. Our social media, emails and videos are wonderful ways to increase our ability to stay connected to many more friends and family around the globe than we ever could before. But they can never be a completely fulfilling substitute for real time human contact, conversation and touch.

Community can come in any form that suits you. Perhaps it is a book club, perhaps a rave. There is volunteering, church or spiritual groups, hiking, cooking, dinner parties, sports, picnics, classes, or mastermind groups. The opportunities are many and as varied as your interests. The fulfillment of authentic communication makes a big difference in engendering happiness and producing energy for other aspects of your life. Party, join, meet, have fun and stay connected to others around you.

I personally need to create a balance between the alone time and social time that my art making and personal and business life require. Yet it is all relationship, one to our inner selves and the other to our outer expression. In our very self-directed goal setting society, discounting the need to take off and celebrate is corrosive of the whole system. Letting go into community and socializing is regenerative.

Pick up your personal and group interactions and see what happens!

STORIES

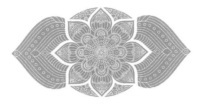

I am an introvert/extrovert combo. Neither is fully satisfying alone. We are all unique combinations of our solo and social worlds. I find that I can stay alone in my garden with all my creative projects for days. When I go out to perform, speak, teach or meet friends I enter the opposite world of socializing. I am astounded at how joyous, expansive and fun it is. Creating a balance is crucial.

Jonathon Bixby

Since I've been teaching dance for more than 30 years, I've seen a lot of people of all ages attempt to learn something new and in particular, swing dancing. Many times, single people have shown up as a way of socializing and meeting new people. Those interactions have often led to romance and marriage.

What I've found fascinating is the transformation that can occur in peoples' confidence levels. The shy ones come out of their shells and socialize by dancing with a stranger. This has been a big step for many. Many women have even learned to ask for the partner they want, reversing dated partner dance rules.

As people age, they seem to drop their inhibitions about everything, especially socializing in the dance arena. I recently received a letter from a woman, thanking me for introducing her to dance. She had put it aside for a while and was now so happy to be back dancing her heart out. She even entered a contest in the 71 year-old category and takes private lessons three times a week![45]

Irene Martinez

My parents came to the USA as war refugees when I was 3 years old. I grew up being told to sit still and be quiet. I have always been shy and introverted, until this past year.

I moved to a new town and entered a relationship within two months of arriving there. It wasn't until the relationship ended that I realized how lonely I was. A long time acquaintance recommended I join a local dance group. She described them as a "fun burlesque fusion dance group of ladies that have a blast dressing up and performing all over town".

I was petrified. I am not a dancer, nor did I consider myself a "social" person or performer. I forced myself to attend the first class. Now, almost a year later, I have performed with them in front of thousands of audience members. I have made hundreds of friends and find myself living in a community of wonderful people who have welcomed and accepted me with open arms. I tell them that I am shy and I am looked at with wide surprised eyes and am told "I don't see that in you."

After feeling like an outsider for the majority of my life and having always been described as a "wall flower", I now finally feel like I belong. It was a year-long process of being surrounded by a group of people who love to perform, socialize and be in the limelight who allowed, encouraged and welcomed my growth from the shy and introverted little girl to the confident and outgoing social butterfly I have transformed into.[46]

SCIENCE

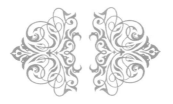

Being members of interdependent groups ensured successful survival for our ancestors. It is in our biology to join together. It is also our deepest natural instinct to know that nothing is separate in ultimate reality or space, as scientists are now discovering and verifying. Everything and everyone is interconnected.[47]

The mental and physical health benefits of having an active social life are many. People who socialize regularly live longer and have a stronger immune system. This creates resilience in maintaining a healthy body throughout life. Interacting with others boosts feelings of well-being and decreases feelings of depression. Research has shown that one sure way of improving your mood is to work on building social connections.[48]

Reports have shown that connecting with others can boost brain health and even help in preventing age-related cognitive disorders like Alzheimer's disease. More recently, there has been accumulating evidence that socializing is good for your mind fitness. People who connect with others generally perform better on tests of memory and other cognitive skills. And in the long run, people with active social lives are less likely to develop dementia than those who are more socially isolated.[49]

Dance is one of the easiest and effective ways to socialize. Its added benefits are agility, balance, flexibility and stamina. It also strengthens bones and cardiovascular systems, while encouraging weight control.[50]

Dance is a visual, socially organized form of communication. It is a vehicle through which group membership and social identity can be expressed. All types of dancers have the potential to identify with one another as sharing in one identity, dancer. Dance can be viewed as an artistic performance or participated in. It can be a career, a form of recreation, or personal self-expression.

There are countless forms and styles of dance. A spectator of a performance learns something about the culture that produced the dance. There is the potential for inter-group contact with a wide variety of dancers and audiences. This can be powerful for changing attitudes and conceptions about different groups. A mind-set expansion can occur as people are exposed to a culture that is presented as art, instead of information via factual accounts such as textbooks.[51] Dance brings unity!

When individual heart energy unites with the coherence of a group, the expanded field adds to the energy and possibility of continuous peace on our planet.

Regardless of how you go about connecting with others, remember to do it in a way that is enjoyable to you, so you will be sure to do it often.

PRACTICES

What are your favorite ways to socialize? Are they quiet like a book club or musical like a swing dance class? Do you like to watch sports with fans of your favorite teams? Or perhaps take a scuba diving or language class, or sing with a friend? Make a list of all the ways you think might be enjoyable for you.

Plan social events ahead on your calendar so the month doesn't fly by without your participation in great celebrations or interactions. Here are some more ideas to gain the benefits of socializing:

1. Volunteer at local charity such as a food bank or homeless shelter.

2. Invite a friend you haven't talked to for a while to coffee or lunch.

3. Use Face Time or Skype to have a "real" visit with friends or relatives from far away.

4. Engage in conversation or just say hello to people you meet during your day.

5. Go to the spiritual center of your choice. In fact, visit a variety of them.

6. Get some exercise in a social way by going to the YMCA or your local gym or club and take any of the many available classes. Take group walks or hikes.

7. Visit your neighborhood or community centers and participate in activities.

8. Go to concerts, museums, art openings or any cultural event that interests you. Ask a friend or go with a group. Or go alone and meet new people!

9. Take a class, learn something new. The Adult Education Centers offer a great variety of choices.

10. If you do not have any in your immediate family, find some children at a local afterschool organization and read to them, help with schoolwork or take for them for an outing.

11. Invite people over for bingo, monopoly, poker or any other board and card games.

12. Sing, dance and make music with others whenever possible.

For longevity and brain health, find social activities that combine both physical and cognitive aspects.

CREATE YOUR OWN PRACTICE

What feels right to me today?

Rest

"Put some space in your pace!"

CHAPTER SEVEN

Rest

GUESS WHAT? IT'S OK TO LET GO and relax! In fact, it is essential on many levels. Downtime allows the pleasure of calm, meditative and receptive states. Most importantly, being relaxed is a brave and innovative approach to life, where we allow our adventure to unfold. This is the opposite of the adrenaline-filled, make-it-happen, forcing approach that we have been conditioned to. Quiet, that rare and undervalued commodity in our over-busy lives, is crucial for experiencing the deep quality of life. It is where rejuvenation on all levels begins. Spaciousness allows the delicious closeness of letting go of all external conditions and checking in with oneself. It is appreciating the beauty of the moment with nowhere to go or anything to do. And it can be as simple as a breath away.

One of the most important concepts when creating vital peace in your life is to be completely fulfilled and appreciative of what is. Slowing down gives you the opportunity to feel this and be grateful for what already is. Expansion grows out of the moment of acknowledging what you already have. Thoughts can then be re-focused to perceiving the next step or direction. Happiness is not based on current circumstances, as life is always in flux. We are powerful creators that can alter our future. Unwanted or past experiences help define new desires but are not permanent conditions. They are more guideposts on the road to expanding our consistent well-being.

Creativity and your unfolding path all happen in empty space, the womb. This is the receptive or feminine mode. It is where you listen, receive information and find your true self and the eternal aspects or basis of life. I do love my lists, but a moment's relief from my own agendas lets me realize the tasks are endless and will never be done. And that is okay. What a fresh concept it is to find strength in allowing emptiness. Everything is created in unfilled room.

Alone time is delectable. Find the meditation practice that pleases you. There are many - from walking to mantra repetition. Rest and nap often; it doesn't mean you are getting old! Give Nature a thumbs up daily. Stop and notice something beautiful around you and get into the wonder of the beauty that is everywhere: the sky, plants, clouds, trees, fragrances. Enjoy relaxing activities. Surrender to the sensual aspects of life. Breathe into what is. Serendipity happens in these states and life becomes easy.

The deepest quality internal relaxation gives is a pervasive serenity, as trust develops in the innately loving and generous nature of life. The peace you find in yourself may be the greatest service that you can give, as we are all connected and it provides this as a basic state and belief for all. Life is on your side, depending on where you habitually place your thoughts. Here all things are possible. So just breathe and know that everything is always working out for the best.

STORIES

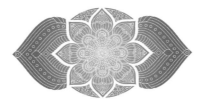

My morning tea ritual is one of my favorite times of day. In this beautiful state between sleeping and waking, it is easy to scan my mind of any blockages to my desires and just sit in the delightful feeling of new possibilities. Thoughts are flowing from this open portal, so I often journal or take notes. In my daily retreat, it is fun to set up the complete enjoyment of each day ahead of it happening.

Jacqui Chandler

I began a mantra-based meditation at the age of 16. I later enrolled in a group meditation practice that participated in an eight week challenge to see if we could impact the local crime rate. We did! So, less than 1% of us tapping into our innate stillness brought us not only personal clarity, but also benefited our community as well.

Today, my meditation practice is in a daily walk, grounding my movement and inner calm with active breathing and mindfulness. Other benefits from meditation that I have noticed are that I let life unfold with less effort. I consciously release accumulated tension back into the flow of life. I sense myself more as a wave of interconnectedness and when a situation triggers an automatic response, I can pause to see how I might trade reaction for thoughtful response.[52]

Paige Kaye

For much of my adult life, I was up at 6:00 am, at the gym by 6:30 and in the office by 8:00 am, wearing my 'work ethic' like a badge of honor. Relaxing was akin to giving up for me. It was the vernacular of luxury and the very idea of it actually had me feeling guilty. My youngest son saw something else though and I can still hear his voice telling me, "Relax Mom." I literally had no way to interpret my son's words into action, I simply had too much to do!

It wasn't until my son left home and I was turning fifty years old that I began to understand the biochemical need to relax, to reduce stress hormones and to slow down the nervous system. Stress, I have now learned, is more often than not self-induced by the mind's belief that we should be able to control our circumstances. Then, almost out of nowhere, relaxing became a calling, a duty to myself that was long overdue. I took a week off and went to a retreat and listened to the ocean and the pines and spent time sitting, walking and slowing down.

Thankfully, I found a new place inside that learned to set to relax mode. Through the practice of noticing breath and thought, I can now tap into a place that I can feel safe in and slowed down, even in the middle of a busy day. I have learned that what I am doing is not as important as who I am being. When I approach the world from a place of not needing anything to be different, it seems to act as a magnet, drawing a world to me that is less hectic and leaves me more alive, refreshed and joyful.[53]

SCIENCE

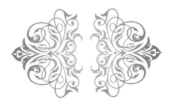

Slowing down the mind and all our physical systems has been proven to be beneficial for every aspect of our lives: health, happiness and success. In this quiet space, clearing takes place and new life is created. Connection to the broadest, multi-dimensional self is given room to blossom. Solutions and creative ideas emerge. Relaxation has many forms: massages, vacationing, walking, listening to music, tub soaking, or whatever allows you to let go and be in an open, empty place. Meditation is also important as a consistent habit for maintaining a peaceful inner life. There are many different techniques; choose one that you feel aligned with and practice regularly for the best results.

Besides the spiritual rewards of relaxation, there are also many health benefits from being in a state of rest. Immune function increases, pain and inflammation decrease. Blood pressure lowers. Stress-related conditions such as depression and anxiety can be alleviated and replaced by positive emotions. Digestion is improved. Blood sugar levels normalize and the activity of stress hormones is reduced. Chronic pains are also lessened.[54]

Many of these conditions listed are communications from the body. Take the time to learn about yourself and what your body wants to tell you. There are underlying mental and emotional causes for your state of health.[55]

When anxieties are lessened, sleep improves. Studies show that the better rested we are, the longer we will live. Being less tired also leads to better sex lives. Resting can help to control weight challenges, as we have more energy to cook and exercise. The body also sends hormonal crave-more-food messages when fatigued.[56]

Meditation improves brain fitness. Scientific research has shown that in the brains of people who meditate often, there is greater volume in the areas of the brain which are related to positive emotions and self-control. They have found that these larger volumes might account for mediators' ability to focus, cultivate positive emotions, retain emotional stability and engage in mindful behavior. Cortical thickness is increased in areas related to paying attention. Quiet time also develops the ability to regulate emotions and improve the ability to introspect, expanding the ability to love yourself. Doing nothing even helps productivity because focus, memory and creativity are increased.[57]

When we are aware of and in control of our own mind's dramas and permutations, we become more compassionate towards others.[58] Regularly choosing and focusing on the positive possibilities for ourselves is deep happiness. Thoughts and emotions create our reality and science says that it is the consciousness of the observer of an experiment that alters the result. Projecting our own positivity into our connected human field of awareness has a profound effect on creating a bright evolution for the future of our planet.

Conditional experience on the outside can't be controlled, but we can direct our lives from the inside with the quality of our thoughts.

PRACTICES

The basic nature of life is dynamic peace. Take a few minutes throughout the day to breathe and enter this state of calm. Setting aside 15 minutes a day to one hour for just quiet time is even better.

Meditate: Meditation has been well documented for its benefits, both physical and mental. There are many methods of meditation.[59] My preference is to sit straight and just breathe in and out, conscious of the air. If a stray thought occurs, I welcome it, enjoy it, let it go and return to my breathing. Since I am a very physical and energetic person, I find that walking will clear my mind and allow new possibilities or dialogue with my inner self. Getting up from my desk and taking a cruise around the neighborhood works wonders. Explore different methods and see what you enjoy, which may change over time.

Breathe: The best thing about using the breath for relaxation is that it is always happening and can be used at any time! Whenever those disconnected-self thoughts or anxieties come in, just stop and take a few deep breaths. It brings you back to your larger, peaceful, non-mental self.

Nature: Stop and praise Nature daily. Take a moment to look at a flower, a mountain, or the lighting on a cloud or a tree. Honor the sun, moon, stars, water, earth and air. Get out daily, even if it is just to your terrace with potted plants. Appreciate the great beauty we are blessed to be part of and live in.

Listen: Take the time to listen to and follow your inner desires.

Imagine: Being quiet and exploring your dreams is a great pleasure and makes them come true.

Sensuality: Touch, smell, taste, savor the essence of being alive.

Travel: Go to places that inspire you, even locally and soak them in.

Gratitude: Take time for appreciation of what is and the gifts to come.

Quiet: Turn off the phone and devices for at least half an hour!

Nap: Rest is powerful.

Do absolutely nothing!

CREATE YOUR OWN PRACTICE

What feels right to me today?

*Thank you for sharing this time
and these ideas with me.*

*Remember, you are spirit in form, love manifest.
Create and enjoy every moment of this great adventure to the fullest!*

Love, Beth

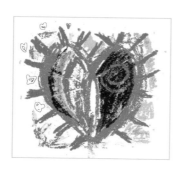

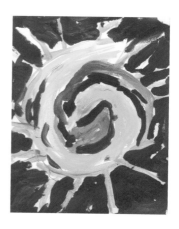

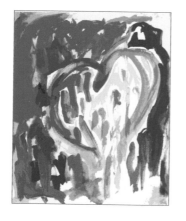

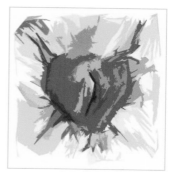

FOOTNOTES, FURTHER READING, AND ACKNOWLEDGMENTS

Chapter 1: Move

[1]Abraham-Hicks:

Daily Quote with Esther Hicks.

www.abraham-hicks.com

Here is the quote that I paraphrased about what success is: "The idea of "success," for most people, revolves around money or the acquisition of property or other possessions, but we consider a state of joy as the greatest achievement of success. And while the attainment of money and wonderful possessions certainly can enhance your state of joy, the achievement of a good-feeling physical body is by far the greatest factor for maintaining a continuing state of joy and well-being. And so, there are few things of greater value than the achievement of a good-feeling body." —Abraham-Hicks

I recommend listening to their YouTube videos as well as reading their materials often. I have found them to be gently balancing and life changing.

[2]Delaney Harding, dance student, Santa Barbara, CA.

[3]Lauren Breese, AIREDANSE, Santa Barbara, CA, www.airedanse.com.

[4]Check out www.joyousmovement.com for videos, class and training information. It is fun dance fitness for every body and ability, and of course, one of my big passions.

[5]Quote is from a staff member at Friendship Center, Montecito, CA. This is an adult day care center for individuals with memory loss at all stages.

[6] Kathryn Eisler Lemay, PhD, Santa Barbara, CA.

[7]Luciana Mitzkun, Dementia Care Specialist, Family Services at Friendship Center and author, Santa Barbara, CA. Her book is *Ahead of Dementia, A Real-World, Upfront, Straightforward, Step-by-Step Guide for Family Caregivers*, Karen Doehner Aldenderfer (ed).

[8]Richard Powers, "Want to Improve Memory? Strengthen Your Synapses. Here's How," (January 8, 2007), https://newswise.com/articles/want-to-improve-memory-strengthen-your-synapses-heres-how.

[9]Richard Powers, "Use It or Lose It: Dancing Makes You Smarter," (July 30, 2010), http://socialdance.stanford.edu/syllabi/smarter.htm. This article includes information from Dr. Joseph Coyle, a Harvard Medical School psychiatrist who wrote an accompanying commentary as well as research from Dr. Katzman who added information on brain fitness.

[10]*Jon Hamilton, "Your Brain's Got Rhythm, And Syncs When You Think,"* (June 17, 2014), http://www.npr.org/sections/health-shots/2014/06/17/322915700/your-brains-got-rhythm-and-syncs-when-you-think. Nathan Urban, a neuroscientist at Carnegie Mellon University in Pittsburgh offers new research on the innate nature of Rhythm in the Body.

[11]Suggested reading: the books of Gregg Braden, Bruce Lipton and Dr. Joe Dispenza. These innovative scientists explore many fascinating and groundbreaking new theories on health, brain chemistry, quantum physics, neuroscience, genetics and human evolution.

[12]Please check out my easy, for absolutely everybody, belly dance videos at www.bethaminebellydance.com. I also have multi-level movement programs on my website: www.joyousmovement.com.

Chapter 2: Nourish

[13]"You are what you eat." This is a quote from Dr. Victor Hugo Lindlahr, an American health food and weight loss pioneer. From 1936 to 1953, he hosted Talks and Diet, a popular radio series about nutrition.

[14]Many informative documentaries are available on food sources and animal farming. If you desire an education on where your food is coming from to help inform you what to eat that is right for you, these are a great resource.

[15]Jatila van der Veen, physics instructor and dancer.
http://web.physics.ucsb.edu/~jatila/
http://jatiladance.com/

[16]Dale Figtree, nutritionist, author of *Delicious, Nutritious and Simple,* (2015). Available on Amazon.com.

[17]Aparna Khanolkar, Ayurvedic lifestyle mentor, chef and author.
http://www.AparnaKhanolkar.com
http://www.amazon.com/author/aparnakhanolkar

[18]Dharma Singh Khalsa, M.D., President and Medical Director of Alzheimer's Research and Prevention Foundation, author of *Food as Medicine.*

http://www.drdharma.com/Public/Bio/FoodasMedicine/index.cfm.

Dharma Singh Khalsa, MD, "Food and Your Health," http://www.drdharma.com/utility/showArticle/?objectID=189.

Dharma Singh Khalsa, MD, "Science Reveals the Anti Aging Benefits of Food," http://www.drdharma.com/utility/showArticle/?objectID=218.

[19]Carol Byrd-Bredbenner, Gaile Moe, Donna Beshgetoor, Jacqueline Berning, *Wardlaw's Perspectives in Nutrition, 9th Edition.*

Carolyn Denton, LN, "How Does Food Impact Health?," University of Minnesota, https://www.takingcharge.csh.umn.edu/explore-healing-practices/food-medicine/how-does-food-impact-health.

[20]Kris Gunnars, BSc, "9 Ways That Processed Foods Are Harming People," (August 1, 2017), https://www.medicalnewstoday.com/articles/318630.php.

[21]Gómez-Pinilla analyzed more than 160 studies about food's effect on the brain. The results of his analysis appear in the July 2008 issue of the journal, *Nature Reviews Neuroscience*, and are available online at www.nature.com/nrn/journal/v9/n7/abs/nrn2421.html.
See also: http://newsroom.ucla.edu/releases/scientists-learn-how-food-affects-52668.

[22]Allison Hodge, "7 Steps to Mindful Eating," One Medical Blog (May 2, 2016), http://www.onemedical.com/blog/live-well/mindful-eating/.

[23]Suggested Reading: Richard Merrill, *The Gardener's Table: A Guide to Natural Vegetable Growing and Cooking*. Available at Amazon.com, this is a comprehensive kitchen garden guide.

Tower Gardens: There are a wide variety of vertical plant growing systems; these are great for small spaces.

Barrel Gardening: Also in a wide variety of styles and are great for growing nutrient rich vegetables in small areas.

Juicing: Juicing is a great way to boost your intake of nutrients. Many styles of juicers are available, find one that is easy to clean and does a great job of extracting.

Chapter 3: Release

[23]There are many methods available for help with identifying and clearing old patterns from the past. Research and find out which techniques feel right to you.

[24]Roxy Angel Superstar, Events Director for the Center of the Heart, Santa Barbara, CA, Roxy is an empath intuitive and author. Reach her at Star Oracle Readings, www.roxyangelsuperstar.com.

[25]Deanna Cohen, Feng Shui Consultant, Santa Barbara, CA.

[26] From Brainworks, Train Your Mind blog: "What are Brainwaves?," http://www.brainworksneurotherapy.com/what-are-brainwaves.

[27]From the Mindvalley Academy blog: "This is How Brain Waves Contribute to the State of Mind," http://www.mindvalleyacademy. com/blog/mind/brain-waves.

[28]Reverend Maryum Morse, Senior Minister, Center of the Heart, Santa Barbara, CA.
www.centeroftheheart.com
email: info@centeroftheheart.com

[29]Greg Braden YouTube video, "How the Heart-Brain Connection Works," https://www.youtube.com/watch?v=6fVwufEZi2Y&sns=em.

[30]Heart Math Institute
https://www.heartmath.org
Science of the Heart: Exploring the Role of the Heart in Human Performance, Heart Math Institute, https://www.heartmath.org/research/ science-of-the-heart/heart-brain-communication/.

[31]Mikael Cho, "How Clutter Affects Your Brain (and What You Can Do About It)," (July 5, 2013), http://www.lifehacker.com/how-clutter-affects-your-brain-and-what-you-can-do-abo-662647035.

[32]Rev. Maryum Morse, Senior Minister, Center of the Heart, Santa Barbara, CA.

[33]Portals to Peace Shrine Making Kits:
www.portalstopeaceshrines.com
Learn about the process of shrine making here, with downloadable shrine booklet.

Chapter 4: Give

[34]Janet Reineck, founder of Dance for Humanity. http://www.worlddanceforhumanity.org

[35]Anaiya Mussolini, Santa Barbara, CA. Anaiya is a cultural philanthropist and adventure enthusiast. She travels the world empowering women through dance and advocating for orphans.
http://www.dancewithanaiya.com
http://www. travelwithanaiya.com

[36]Scott Bea, PsyD, "Wanna Give? This Is Your Brain on a 'Helper's High," (November 15, 2016), https://health.clevelandclinic.org/2016/11/why-giving-is-good-for-your-health/ 2016.

[37]From the HeartMath Institute, Expanding Heart Connections Blog: "The Energetic Heart is Unfolding," with excerpts from "The Energetic Heart: Bioelectromagnetic Communication Within and Between People" by HeartMath Director of Research, Rollin McRaty, (July 22, 2010), https://www.heartmath.org/articles-of-the-heart/science-of-the-heart/the-energetic-heart-is-unfolding.

[38]Greg Braden, YouTube videos: "How The Heart-Brain Connection Works," https://youtu.be/6fVwufEZi2Y.
"Heart Mind Coherence," https://youtu.be/iYRtFt2UTOA.
"Greg Braden on the Magnetic Field of the Heart," https://youtu.be/ PauUWFSGNVA.

Chapter 5: Create

[39]Shannon Jaffee, Teacher, Santa Barbara, CA.

[40]Seyburn Zorthian, www.seyburnzorthian.com, Santa Barbara, CA.

[41]James Clear, "Make More Art: The Health Benefits of Creativity, (December 23, 2015), http://www.huffingtonpost.com/james-clear/make-more-art-the-health-benefits-of-creativity_b_8868802.html.

[42]From the Lillstreet Art Center Blog: "7 Ways We Benefit From Creativity," https://lillstreet.com/7benefitsofcreativity.

[43]Richard Powers, "Use it or Lose It: Dancing Makes You Smarter, Longer," (July 30, 2010), https://socialdance.stanford.edu/syllabi/smarter.htm.

[44]New Realities Interview with Dr. Joe Dispenza: "Creativity and the Unknown," https://www.youtube.com/watch?v=uz5QI0vxOsc&sns=em.

Chapter 6: Join

[45]Jonathon Bixby, www.dancesantabarbara.com, Santa Barbara, CA.

[46]Irene Martinez, Psychologist, Santa Barbara, CA.

[47]From the One Mind–One Energy, The Power is Within blog: "Are We All Connected?," http://www.one-mind-one-energy.com/connected.html.

[48] Angela K. Troyer PhD, CPsych, "The Health Benefits of Socializing," *Psychology Today* (June 30, 2016), https://www.psychologytoday.com/blog/living-mild-cognitive-impairment/201606/the-health-benefits-socializing.

[49]TAngela K. Troyer PhD, CPsych, "The Health Benefits of Socializing," *Psychology Today* (June 30, 2016), https://www.psychologytoday.com/blog/living-mild-cognitive-impairment/201606/the-health-benefits-socializing.

[50]Enjoydance.com, "Benefits of Dancing," http://www.enjoydance.com/benefits-of-dancing.html.

[51]From an article written by Rachyl Pines and Howard Giles from the University of California at Santa Barbara.

Pines, R., & Giles, H. (in press). "Dance and intergroup communication." In H. Giles & J. Harwood (Eds.), Oxford Encyclopedia of Intergroup Communication. New York, NY: Oxford University Press.

Rachyl Pines: rpines@umail.ucsb.edu
Howard Giles: giles@comm.ucsb.edu.

Chapter 7: Relax

[52]Jacquie Chandler, www.sustaintahoe.org, sustaintahoe@gmail.com.

[53]Paige Kaye, Realtor, www.paigekaye.com, Santa Barbara, CA.

[54]Mayo Clinic Staff, "Relaxation techniques: Try these steps to reduce stress," (April 19, 2017), https://www.mayoclinic.org/healthy-lifestyle/stress-management/in-depth/relaxation-technique/art-20045368.

[55]Louise Hay, founder of Hay House Publishing and author of *You Can Heal Your Life*.

[56]R. Morgan Griffin, "9 Surprising Reasons to Get More Sleep," (December 27, 2011), https://www.webmd.com/sleep-disorders/features/9-reasons-to-sleep-more#2.

[57]Emma M. Seppälä, PhD, "20 Scientific Reasons to Start Meditating Today," (September 11, 2013), https://www.psychologytoday.com/blog/feeling-it/201309/20-scientific-reasons-start-meditating-today.

[58]Alyssa Sparacino, "11 Surprising Health Benefits of Sleep," (July 21, 2013), http://www.health.com/health/gallery/0,,20459221,00.html#ad-3.

[59]Meghan Greene, "7 Types of Meditation: Which One Is Best for You?," (February 5, 2015), https://visualmeditation.co/7-types-of-meditation/.

THE ART OF A HAPPY LIFE

1. Dance and move your body. This is essential.

2. Enjoy growth and expansion. Life is a fluid state.

3. Eat a plant based diet, organic when possible.

4. Forgive the past.

5. Expand kindness every day, even if it is one smile. This exchange enlarges the spirit and feels good.

6. Enjoy the uncertainty of living; it is a journey of transformative adventure.

7. Follow your inner desires, and take the time to listen.

8. Vision your good, the life you would love to lead.

9. Trust in life, as its nature is love. It is on your side, depending on where you habitually place your thoughts.

10. Acknowledge yourself often as a reflection of the wonder and beauty of being alive. You are made of the earth and the stars.

11. Put some space in your pace. Continuous rushing is wearing on the soul.

12. Stop and praise Nature daily. It can be as simple as a moment to look at a flower, a mountain, or the lighting on a tree.

13. Find the humor and the positive in most situations.

14. Enjoy the sensual wonder of being alive now.

15. Remember that happiness is a choice and life is meant to be fun!

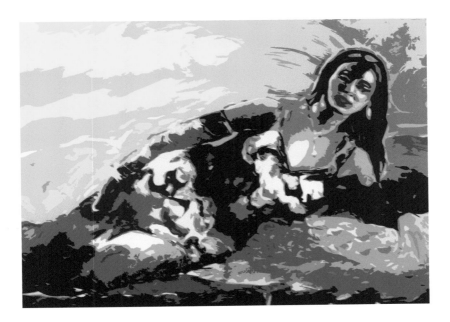

All paintings and quotes are by Beth Amine.

**Other Beth Amine products and websites
for your personal pleasure:**

www.joyouseverydayliving.com

www.joyousmovement.com

www.bethaminebellydance.com

www.portalstopeaceshrines.com

www.whenbrushesdance.com

www.bethamine.com

CPSIA information can be obtained at www.ICGtesting.com
Printed in the USA
BVIW12n2030210118
505481BV00001B/1

* 9 7 8 1 9 7 9 8 5 3 4 5 3 *